Sociology, Nursing and Health

WITHDRAWN

Sociology, Nursing and Health

Anne Williams
BA MA PhD RGN RM

Professor of Nursing, School of Health Science, University of Wales, Swansea

Hannah Cooke
BSc MSc(Econ) MSc RGN NDN RNT

Lecturer in Nursing, University of Manchester School of Nursing Studies, Manchester

Carl May
BSc Econ(Wales) PhD(Edin)

Senior Research Fellow, Department of General Practice, University of Manchester, Manchester

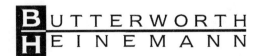

OXFORD   BOSTON   JOHANNESBURG   MELBOURNE   NEW DELHI   SINGAPORE

Butterworth-Heinemann
Linacre House, Jordan Hill, Oxford OX2 8DP
225 Wildwood Avenue, Woburn, MA 01801-2041
A division of Reed Educational and Professional Publishing Ltd

A member of the Reed Elsevier plc group

First published 1998

British Library Cataloguing in Publication Data
A catalogue record for this book is available from the British Library

Library of Congress Cataloguing in Publication Data
A catalogue record for this book is available from the Library of Congress

ISBN 0 7506 3619 X

Typeset by ✒ Tek-Art, Croydon, Surrey
Printed in Great Britain by Biddles Ltd., Guildford and King's Lynn

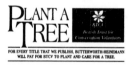

Contents

Foreword

The topic of health has been high on the political agenda for the past decade and looks likely to remain so. It has been a turbulent time for health professionals. Changes are taking place when there are serious problems of morale within the whole arena of health care. Essentially these problems are caused by pressure on resources, both financial and human. Attempts to control the soaring costs of health care have affected every single aspect of the NHS. At the same time the extent of change and the number of changes have been remarkable, fundamentally altering the nature of the health service. Crucially, however, attempts to improve the quality of health service need to be buttressed by changes in training and education.

The variety of occupations involved in health care is tremendous and each occupation needs to develop its own sound body of knowledge. Each group brings different skills and different solutions to the health care problem with which they are presented. However, there is a more fundamental overview on health which needs to be confronted and this volume provides the goods by unashamedly announcing the importance of the sociological approach in studying health.

Among sociologists, concern with health and illness is comparatively recent. Even after the Second World War, the sociology of medicine was very slow to develop. However, the past decade has been an important period in the examination of health problems. Probably the most important contributions of sociologists in this field have been to provide fresh insights that implicitly challenge traditional medical assumptions. The crucial shift, which occurred towards the end of the 1970s, was the recognition that sociologists should be concerned with issues of health and illness rather than medicine. This helped to create the idea that the emphasis should be towards being more patient-oriented than doctor-oriented. Sociologists set down the gauntlet by reminding us that what is in the interests of the doctor may not always be equally in the interests of the patient. However, the facts cannot be ignored. The dominant occupation in the provision of health care continues to be the medical profession. In contrast, in seeking to gain in occupational status, nursing is facing an uphill struggle.

Some of the hopes of those applauding the vision underpinning the radical proposals known as Project 2000, agreed by the UKCC in 1985 but only later supported by the government, have not yet come fully to fruition. Health professionals, and nurses in particular, need to embrace a wider perspective than hands-on skills. The need is an urgent one. Currently, within the NHS, the group which is increasingly affecting the occupational strategies of doctors and nurses is that of *management*. Following the introduction of general management in the 1980s, nursing lost its right to have a place at the top management level of health care. This loss may have been important in affecting occupational power. Furthermore, the organizational changes in the 1990s have not favoured nursing. An important response is to improve the eduction of nurses.

This book exemplifies the way that health professionals can most usefully gain an understanding of health and health care. More specifically, it illuminates the relationship between nursing and sociology. I was first introduced to the approach underpinning this book as external examiner to the nursing degree at Manchester. In developing an appreciation of sociological insights, there was no attempt to 'speak down' to students; students gained in confidence as they themselves embraced sociological ideas. I was amazed at what could be accomplished by excellent teaching. The approach has now been successfully transferred to one volume. The book provides an important education.

Keith Soothill
Professor of Social Research
Lancaster University

Introduction

What is sociology and why is it relevant to nursing?

When working in a college of nursing in the 1980s, one of the authors taught the six-week introductory block for RGN students. Among all the anatomy and physiology, blood pressures and bed bathing, students were required to meet a learning objective which stated that they would 'understand the nature of man' by the end of the block. Never mind the fact that social scientists and philosophers have been grappling with this problem for centuries, these nursing students would know the answer in a few short weeks.

Happily, nurse education has moved on a little since this time. It does not expect to have all the answers and to impart them neatly packaged to students. While it is tempting to try to define human nature and to have one neat, tidy answer to the human nature question, this is a temptation we should resist. Cowen (1994) suggests that the assertion that something is 'just human nature' or that 'you can't change human nature' is frequently summoned to clinch an argument, to have the last word on the subject. It is an argument used to justify the status quo and fend off demands for change. He gives us an example of the boxing champion defending his sport on the grounds that is it 'just human nature'. Our beliefs about human nature have, however, changed as the historical context has changed. The answer we give to this question today is different from answers given in the past, and arguably from answers that will be given in the future. Two hundred years ago the spectator who enjoyed cock fighting or bear baiting probably argued that it was 'just human nature'. Today the computer is often used as a metaphor for the human mind, but will we make such comparisons in future centuries when computer technology seems old fashioned?

Theories of human nature have always played a key role in political movements and have been used to justify political changes. Social Darwinism, for example, played a vital role in justifying the genocidal policies of the Nazis. In the 1980s individualistic conceptions of human nature played an important role in the creation of the 'enterprise culture'. These ideas justified cuts in welfare services in the interests of 'individual self reliance'. Cowen suggests that the phrase 'you can't change human nature' is a prescription not a truth. It is a device used to close down debate and to stifle possibilities of change.

If there is no universal definition of human nature then, similarly there is no universally accepted definition of nursing, despite the best efforts of nursing theorists. Our ideas about nursing are situated in a particular social and historical context and we need to understand the way in which that changing context influences our current conceptions of our occupation. While definitions of nursing are not fixed and immutable, we may be prepared to acknowledge that nursing is an occupation which involves human beings, their actual or potential health problems and some kind of helping role on the part of the nurse. Such an occupation necessarily draws on knowledge from a variety of subjects such as biology, sociology, psychology, politics and ethics. Nursing has drawn heavily on sociology to inform its own ideas and theories about nursing. Concepts, such as role, interaction, stress and bureaucracy all derive at least in part from sociological work. Nurse theorists have not always been prepared to acknowledge such borrowing.

Sociology, to state the obvious, is engaged in the study of human societies. Sociologists are concerned with understanding society in a 'disciplined' way (Berger 1966) involving both a theoretical understanding of social issues and empirical investigation bound by explicit rules of evidence. Sociology arose out of the 'two great revolutions' in Europe. It arose as Europeans strove to understand the enormous social changes that confronted them and tried to anticipate their consequences (Giddens 1986).

By its very nature, sociology deals with issues that are very pressing to us all. It confronts problems which are often subjects of major controversy in society, such as the relationship between social class and illness, the changing role of religion, the rising divorce rate and the changing nature of work. Perhaps because of its subject matter, sociology 'raises hackles that other academic subjects fail to reach' (Giddens 1995, p.18). Maybe because we all have our own cherished views on such controversial topics, sociology is often derided as 'obscure' and 'jargon ridden' (What do you get when you cross a sociologist with a Mafiosi? An offer you can't understand (Giddens 1995, p.19)), and yet if we agree with its premises it is 'just common sense'.

Sociology may also be seen as subversive. Sharp (1995) is 'alarmed' that in encouraging nurses to be critical and questioning 'sociology might stir student nurses into some form of revolutionary praxis' (p.54). Giddens argues that sociologists must not shy away from controversy. If sociologists are not prepared to confront the major social issues of their day, their work becomes merely pointless armchair theorizing. According to Giddens: 'More than any other intellectual endeavour, sociological reflection is central to grasping the social forces remaking our lives today. Social life has become episodic, fragmentary and dogged with new uncertainties which it must be the business of creative sociologists to help us understand better' (Giddens 1995, p.20).

It has been argued that sociology lacks the certainty and precision of the natural sciences. A variety of different theoretical perspectives compete for supremacy. This has led to the subject being regarded as less 'scientific' than the natural sciences in some quarters. Sharp (1995) has argued that sociology is of little value to nurses because it contains diverse points of view and therefore it cannot offer a 'prescription for action'. In the first place this view overestimates the unity of perspective within the natural sciences (e.g. see Davey (1992), for a discussion of the debates within the biological sciences). Secondly, Sharp shows a remarkably facile view of the nature of nursing. Sharp's nurses need to be told what to do, they do not need to be able to think for themselves.

Giddens says that sociology 'does not come neatly gift wrapped, making no demands except that its contents be unpacked' (1986, p.2). Sharp thinks that it is therefore a much too difficult and confusing subject for nurses. Nursing, according to Sharp, should confine its attention to 'instrumental knowledge' and avoid disciplines like sociology which encourage reflection, scepticism and uncertainty.

It is hard to imagine many circumstances in which instrumental knowledge alone would suffice in guiding nurses through their everyday work. A nurse recently recalled the day that a young woman arrested and died on her ward in the presence of her two young children. Another tells of the dilemmas of caring for an end-stage renal failure patient whose dialysis has been discontinued. Another recounts the strains of dealing with parasuicide patients in an environment where hostile and negative attitudes to such patients prevail. A nurse tells of the daily dilemmas of trying to care for groups of patients while knowing that a heavy workload means that hospital rules and procedures cannot be complied with. What 'prescription for action' can we offer these nurses from either the biological or the social sciences? The answer is none. However, we can help the nurse to understand these situations better, in order to make more informed and thoughtful decisions.

Giddens argues that the presence of diverse theoretical perspectives in sociology is a strength, because it 'accurately gives voice to the pluralism that must exist when one studies something so complex and controversial as human social behaviour and institutions' (Giddens, 1995 p.19). Robinson (1992) suggests that this pluralism is of particular value to nurses, because occupational groups are often poor at questioning the assumptions and terms of reference of their own discipline.

C. Wright Mills (1959) used the term the 'sociological imagination' to describe the 'promise' of sociology. For Mills 'the sociological imagination enables us to grasp history and biography and the relations between the two in society. That is its task and its promise.' (p.12) Mills explains this in terms of the relationship between private 'troubles' and public 'issues'. 'Troubles' occur within the lives of individuals and their immediate social world. 'Issues' transcend the individual and have to do with public institutions and the larger structures of social and historical life. Illness is a very private trouble and yet a very public issue – not least because of the social causes of much ill health and premature death. The individual dying of lung cancer faces a very personal tragedy, and yet this is also a public matter as the recent debates on tobacco advertising and sponsorship have emphasized.

Sociological enquiry can illuminate and help make sense of the relationship between private troubles and public issues. Sometimes sociological studies will provide evidence which seems at odds with our common-sense understanding of an issue. Sociology can help us to question our beliefs by presenting us with empirical data which challenges the orthodox view of an issue. For example, Blaxter (1990) found that despite all the attention paid to the effect of healthy and unhealthy behaviours such as diet, exercise and smoking on health, socioeconomic circumstances carried more weight. While healthy behaviours improved the health of the advantaged, they made little impression on the health of the disadvantaged. Unhealthy behaviour did not reinforce disadvantage to the same extent that healthy behaviour increased the advantages of the better off. If we take this data seriously, then income distribution and working conditions become even more important public health issues than smoking habits or diet.

Giddens (1986) says that the sociological imagination should involve an historical, an anthropological and a critical sensitivity. The sociological imagination is historical in that it allows us to understand the distinctive nature of our present society by comparing it with the past. It allows us to see the 'kaleidoscope' of different forms of social life that exist in the world. These two dimensions lead us to the third dimension of 'critical sensitivity'. The sociological imagination shows us that existing social relations are not fixed and immutable and thus it expands our consciousness of the different possibilities for the future which are open to us (Cooke 1993).

Sociology can thus be of value to nurses to enable us to question the values and beliefs of our occupation and the organizational context in which we work. Critique and questioning must be based on analysis and supported by evidence. We need to understand the social forces which shape and constrain our lives in order to change them. Giddens suggests that we need to 'break free of the straitjacket of thinking only in terms of the type of society we know in the here and now' (1986, p.22) and imagine new futures for ourselves.

According to Giddens, no social processes are unalterable laws, and as human beings we are not 'condemned to be swept along by forces that have the inevitability of laws of nature' (1986, p.22). As nursing is swept along by the tide of rapid change in society and in health care we can turn to the sociological imagination to help us to understand what is happening to us. Sociology can help us to take a hand in controlling our own destinies.

Purpose of the book and its main themes

The purpose of the book is to provide readers with a guide to some of the classic and contemporary sociological debates which influence understandings of health and health care – most particularly the practice of nursing – rather than to present a comprehensive overview of sociology as applied to nursing and health care.

The relevant sociology literature is wide-ranging and includes a number of specialist substantive areas, for example family, work, professions and professionalization, conceptions of health and illness, to name but a few of the areas. The literature also includes debates about the nature of knowledge including sociological knowledge, and accounts of classical and contemporary sociologists' contributions to the discipline and to scholarship more generally. We attempt to chart a course through such literature in a way that is meaningful for nurses as well as others involved in health care. We hope that readers will be encouraged to explore the wide sociology literature upon which we draw and, based on their own experiences of providing care, to look critically at sociological ideas that are used to explore and explain health issues.

The core of the book falls into two major sections: Part One, 'Understanding the Social Context of Care', provides a discussion of aspects of the context within which nurses and others who provide care practise. The chapters within this section look critically at some of the taken-for-granted components of everyday life. Discussion includes a review of the dynamics of society. We then look at the breadth and diversity of sociological ideas about family and community, noting their relevance for health and health care. The final chapter in this section explores sociological studies of religions and their application to health and health care. In each chapter you will find reference to how founding sociologists such as Durkheim, Weber and Marx have shaped ideas and prompted debates which have been taken up by contemporary sociologists. We also draw on social commentators from other disciplines, perhaps most obviously social anthropology, as boundaries between disciplinary spheres of knowledge about society, family, community and religion are not clear cut.

Part Two, 'Sociological Perspectives on Nursing and Health', opens with a discussion of the work of nursing and its relationship to wider changes in work and work organization in society. In the chapter which follows, we turn our attention towards the patient as the focus for nursing work and knowledge, suggesting that nursing goes beyond focusing on disease and pathology to incorporate a much wider definition of both ill-health and personhood. This discussion is followed by a consideration of lay and professional perspectives on ill-health and how ill-health is experienced. Finally, we comment on death and its denial which, we suggest, brings us back to the beginning of the book where we observe how society is, fundamentally, a response to the overwhelming inevitability of 'natural' events.

A key message for readers is this: as nurses and others who practise health care, we are critically involved in making sense and giving purpose to life, illness and death. Drawing on ideas we hold in common, we construct versions of each which will have an impact on those we encounter in our practice. At the same time, we are subject to the constructions of others who shape our professional destiny; policy makers and other professionals perhaps most notably medical. Power is a key factor at play in the processes of interplay between, on the one hand, action and agency and, on the other, the factors, structural and otherwise which constrain. We look at the issue of power in some detail throughout the book. The ethical component of such processes should not be ignored, and we take as our starting point in this respect the words of Durkheim who observes that ethics is a function of social organization and as such is embroiled in the puzzles and perplexities of everyday relationships (Durkheim as quoted by Richter 1961, p.182).

There are many themes of sociological and nursing interest contained within the covers of this book. We would like to draw readers' attention to two interlinked themes which we see as central to our project which is to illuminate the relationship between nursing and sociology, and associated issues. The themes are as follows: first, the sociological critique of individualism and, second, 'inequality' as a critique of 'difference'. Within each theme it is possible to identify ideas and issues which have become the currency of sociological thinking and debate and which have infiltrated the languages of nursing and health care. We briefly identify ideas and issues around, for example, social context and power; structural variables such as class, gender and race; as well as morality, identity and politics within the following discussion. These are explored in detail within the remaining chapters together with other ideas and issues of central importance to nursing and sociology. Clearly, there will be themes which we do not emphasize and which readers may consider important. Thus readers will, we hope, engage in the process of critique which this book is intended to foster.

Sociology as a critique of individualism

Hughes, Martin and Sharrock (1995, p.7) make the point that 'it is not too much of a distortion to describe the rise of sociology as part of a reaction against the individualism so prominently displayed in the thought of the enlightenment during the seventeenth and eighteenth centuries'. They go on to remind us, however, that the task of sociology is 'not so much to eliminate the individual as a focus of intellectual attention as to find a way of understanding the relationship between the individual and society' (p.10). Throughout the book we aim to show how sociologists have assisted an understanding of this relationship and to assess its relevance for nursing and health care. In chaper 1, 'Society', we look at how classical sociologists have pursued such an understanding. We note how this sociological project continues in the wake of the influence of enlightenment thinking on contemporary economics and politics. In Chapter 2, 'The Family', we comment on individualistic explanations of family health status, showing how blaming 'individuals' and 'individual' families for behaviours which promote their ill-health (e.g. poor nutrition, smoking and so on) is a device which has been used by health policy makers who appear to ignore the sociological point which is that social and psychosocial contextual factors play an important part in influencing healthy lifestyles and behaviours. Factors such as class, age, location, race and gender, which may affect one's access to resources, are important in evaluating health status.

In Chapter 3, we note how the idea of community has been romanticized by sociologists. And it is interesting to consider how this romanticism appears to have stemmed, at least in part, from a sense of loss of genuine community in the wake of the increasing individualism of the new industrial order of nineteenth century capitalist modes of production. As indicated in Chapter 4, religion is a useful focus for considering the tension between the freely acting individual and a constraining society within the context of health and health care. The chapter also identifies notions of individual responsibility for ill-health *vis* social causes. Discussion in Chapter 5, 'Nursing and working', contains a clear refutation of the individualist credo as it applies to health work. Here we discuss the ownership of emotions and the questions raised include not only whether or not nursing involves emotional labour but also who controls it and who benefits from it?

In Chapter 6, 'The nurse and the patient', context is highlighted in a discussion of nurse–patient interactions and the theme of context is elaborated from a slightly different perspective in the following chapter which deals with lay and professional perspectives on ill-health where, it is argued, health and ill-health are best seen not as objective categories but as 'fundamentally social states of affairs' (Turner 1995). In other words, our very ideas about what ill-health is are the product of interactions that take place within those relationships. The point is made that sociology seeks to understand the social and historical contexts within which interactions occur. Such an understanding opens the way to explorations of the exercise of power, particularly medical power. It also takes us into the realm of social constructionism and the dynamics of identity – construction of boundaries between 'us' and 'them', 'self' and 'other', 'deviant' and 'non-deviant' and so on. These themes are raised in Chapter 1 and revisited in various guises throughout the book.

Our explorations of the sociological critique of individualism continue into the last chapter of the book where we show how sociologists have challenged rationalist scientific medico-legal discourses of death, showing them to be not only individualistic but also masculinist. We end the book with a reference to the 'high cost of dying' and medicolegal debates about whether individual lives are worth living. This takes us back to the beginning of the book, Chapter 1, where we commence with a quote from Berger (1967): 'every human society is in the last resort men (and women) banded together in the face of death'. What we hope to underline throughout our discussions is that what we face is not merely the onslaught of nature but the full force of culture, particularly in the sense of prevailing ideologies which promote selfishness and which undermine a healthy society.

Inequalities vis differences in health

From an individualist perspective, we make 'choices' about lifestyle and behaviours related to health. From this perspective, we might expect that behaviours matter in health, and much of health work tends to be premised on the notion that if one changes one's unhealthy behaviour, health will follow. Set against this perspective are generalizations about class as an indicator of health status; for example, those in non-manual classes enjoy better health than those in manual classes and that the health of those in the North of the UK is worse than those who live in the South. As Blaxter (1990, p.203) suggests, both positions are correct in certain circumstances and yet both provide a limited analysis. She observes that 'the simple question – which is the more important, the environment or the behaviour? – is probably impossible to answer'. However, she goes on to suggest that health is clearly patterned by social class and she asks if it is possible to estimate how much of this effect is due to economic circumstances, and how much to 'voluntary' lifestyles? How protective is 'healthy behaviour, if circumstances are unfavourable?' (p.204).

Blaxter provides a careful exploration of these questions through the health and lifestyle survey, examining behaviours which include, for example, smoking, diet and exercise across social classes and in relation to geographical location. She comes to the tentative conclusion that 'behavioural habits are certainly relevant to health, but perhaps less so than the social environment in which they are embedded' (p.202). As we point out in the previous section of this introduction to the book, she concludes that unhealthy behaviour does not reinforce disadvantage to the same extent as healthy behaviour increases advantage (p.233). The implication of this conclusion, as she later writes, is that 'health policies which focus on the individual may be ineffective not only because exposure to health risks is largely involuntary, but also (as her study shows) because of unwarrented assumptions about the extent to which behaviour can, in these (disadvantaged) circumstances, be effective in improving health' (Blaxter 1990, p.243).

A key aspect of Blaxter's analysis is that from a sociological perspective – one which focuses on context, '**differences** in health are not the same as **inequalities**' (p.237 [the latter is our emphasis]). 'Difference' is an idea available to, and used by, both those who uphold individualism and by those who challenge it. However, difference is used in a particular way by the former to justify policies which aim to change behaviour, placing the responsibility for change on the individual. The sociological critique of this position as illustrated by Blaxter is to emphasize 'probabilities, on the likelihood of good or bad health' which 'focuses attention on the way in which it is the **expectation** [our emphasis] of good or poor health which is unequal' (p.237). In short, one's class position (as well as other factors such as race and gender) is importantly related to health status, although the relationship is not simple and straightforward. It is from this broadly sociological perspective that we explore inequalities within this book. For example, in Chapter 2 we look briefly at the Marxist critique of the family as a central institution in the reproduction of class inequalities. We then turn to feminist critiques which emphasize how the family not only serves to perpetuate class but also gender inequalities. In Chapter 3, we explore inequalities in health in the community. And as we are reminded in Chapter 5 in relation to the work of nursing, structured inequalities in society largely centre around a person's status in their paid work. In Chapter 7, we see that professional and lay discourses on ill-health are profoundly affected by the social and historical contexts in which they are located, including an economic and political system which relies on personal moral responsibility for individual prosperity and self actualization (Lupton 1995). The relationships between lay and professional notions of ill-health are powerfully influenced by the structural variables of gender, class, ethnicity and age.

From one perspective, the sociological critique of difference and the focus on 'inequalities' constitutes an important intellectual contribution to understanding health and health care. It is also a strongly political and moral standpoint. In the various writings on which we draw, we find that sociologists have a view about how things ought to be which infuses their work (readers will note the same applies to the authors of this book). In relation to the current discussion of inequalities, it is useful to consider what might constitute a sociological response to the problem of how do we create a more healthy society.

Wilkinson (1996) proposes that there are compelling arguments to support a collective, social and cohesive approach to dealing with overcoming health inequalities. Such a position is, he argues, in stark contrast to what he describes as a 'cash and keys' society in which cash equips us to take part in transactions mediated by the market, while keys protect us from each other's envy and greed' (p.226). Wilkinson comments on how instead of being people who share social bonds and common interests, 'others' have become 'rivals, competitors for jobs, for houses, space, seats on the bus, parking places', added to which are 'processes of social comparison . . . everything is constantly monitored'. He goes on to suggest that 'there can be no doubt that economic systems that destroy a spirit of social cooperation may incur very high additional costs as a result' (p.229).

Wilkinson (1996, p.221) suggests we try to effect less inequality in health through a social cohesion model. He (Wilkinson 1996, p.221) refers to Putnum and the concept of social capital:

> 'Social capital' . . . features of social life – networks, norms, and trust – that
> enable participants to act together more effectively to pursue shared objectives
> . . .. To the extent that the norms, networks and trust link substantial sectors of
> the community and span underlying social cleavages – to the extent that the
> social capital is of a bridging sort – then the enhanced cooperation is likely to
> serve broader interests and to be widely welcomed.
>
> (Putnam as quoted by Wilkinson 1996, p.221)

Readers will have their various views on the feasibility of such a standpoint for developing healthy societies. Wilkinson draws on a number of examples to support the possibility, not least Titmuss's (1970) *The Gift Relationship: from human blood to social policy*. Titmuss compared and contrasted the US and the UK systems for collecting blood for transfusion. In Britain there was no commercial market in blood, while in the US, blood was increasingly collected by profit-making blood banks, including monopoly rights to collect blood from prisons. Setting aside the possibility that poor quality blood might result from a system of collection that inevitably attracted 'skid row' donors with the possibility of infection with hepatitis, veneral disease and jaundice, the main point of Titmuss's argument according to Wilkinson is that:

> A non-commercial health service which provided patients with medical care and blood freely as they needed it, elicited a willingness amongst the public to make entirely voluntary donations of blood to unknown recipients on a scale large enough to meet society's blood needs. (About one third of the eligible population were donors)
>
> (Wilkinson 1996, pp.227–228)

Wilkinson presses the point that systems which permit and elicit voluntary giving not only create opportunities for people to express themselves through altruism and public spiritness, but also help to create a kind of cohesive moral community. Wilkinson's overall thesis is that increasing inequality imposes a psychological burden which reduces the well-being of society. The resolution of this situation, however, does not mean choosing between greater equity and economic growth. Rather, he suggests that investment in social capital increases efficiency.

For some readers, Wilkinson's work here may appear to be an argument which could be extended to support strategies to utilize a volunteer workforce in order to save costs of running an increasingly expensive health service. This could be seen as exploitation or it could be seen as offering flexibility. As nurses, we are familiar with ambiguities around the justification of work organization. We ourselves are aware of the current tensions between, on the one hand, a concern for the common good and the welfare of our patients and clients – of working in partnership with them – and, on the other hand, the need to preserve a sense of self-identity in our interactions. We are aware of the pull between cooperating with other professional groups and the need to maintain a sense of professional identity (Williams, Robins and Sibbald 1997). We daily reconcile the ideas of care, compassion and engagement with the ideas of objectivity, detachment and competition as indeed do other healthcare professionals. One possible sociological message is that an imbalance in favour of the latter set of ideas (objectivity, detachment and competition) leads to societies which are morally bankrupt and within which lack of cooperation and social cohesion makes for inefficiency.

Reading this book

This book can be read in a number of ways. It contains a number of chapters – essays which address ideas, issues and processes of concern to nurses and others interested in the healthcare field. In doing this it is unlike many similar texts (written mainly for doctors and students of medicine or for 'medical' sociologists) whose authors appear to believe that hospitals are run by doctors. It brings nursing and nurses centrally into the debates.

Readers are invited to 'dip into' the pages of this book according to their nursing and health interests. For example, some will prefer to go directly to Part Two, and to the chapters which deal most directly with lay/professional perspectives on health and patient–nurse relationships. For those approaching the relevance of sociology to nursing and health for the first time, the book provides a discussion of key issues and a guide to further reading within the references. Many readers may wish to consider how specific topics (e.g. family, community, religion or death) are treated in this book as compared with other texts.

As well as demonstrating the sociological contribution to health and nursing, the book also says something about sociology and its practice and will be of interest to some readers specifically for this reason. Importantly, it is a book which comments on the relationship between nursing and sociology. To this end, and to reiterate the point made earlier, we encourage readers to consider the validity and relevance of the sociological accounts of processes with which they will be familiar insofar as they practise nursing and health care. It is important that as nurses we look critically at the disciplines upon which we draw.

Finally, It has been our intention in writing this book to reduce the invisibility of nurses in sociological accounts of health and illness. Perhaps we have not gone far enough in this respect. It is the readership which will judge how far this is the case. It is hoped that the book will at the very least prompt further discussions and further accounts in this respect.

References

Berger P. (1966) *Invitation to Sociology.* Harmondsworth, Middlesex, Penguin.

Berger P. (1967) *The Sacred Canopy: elements of a sociological theory of religion.* New York, Doubleday.

Blaxter M. (1990) *Health and Lifestyles.* London, Routledge.

Cooke H. (1993) Why teach sociology. *Nurse Education Today* 13, 210–216.

Cowen H. (1994) *The Human Nature Debate: social theory, social policy and the caring professions.* London, Pluto.

Davey B. (1992) Biological perspectives in Robinson K. and Vaughan B. (eds) *Knowledge for Nursing Practice.* Oxford, Butterworth-Heinemann.

Giddens A. (1986) *Sociology: a brief but critical introduction* 2nd edn. London, Macmillan.

Giddens A. (1995) In defence of sociology. *New Statesman and Society* 7the April.

Hughes J., Martin P. and Sharrock W. (1995) *Understanding Classical Sociology.* London, Sage.

Lupton D. (1995) *Medicine as Culture: illness, disease and the body in western societies.* London, Sage.

Mills C. Wright (1959) *The Sociological Imagination.* New York, Oxford University Press.

Putnam R.D. (1995) Tuning in, tuning out: the strange disappearance of social capital in America. *Political Science and Politics* December 664–683.

Richter M. (1964) Durkheim's politics and political theory, in Wolff K. (ed.) *Essays on Sociology and Philosophy by E. Durkheim et al.* New York, Harper Torch Books.

Robinson K. (1992) Sociological perspectives, in Robinson K. and Vaughan B. (eds) *Knowledge for Nursing Practice.* Oxford, Butterworth-Heinemann.

Sharp K. (1995) Why indeed should we teach sociology? A response to Hannah Cooke *Nurse Education Today* 15, 52–55.

Titmuss R.M. (1970) *The Gift Relationship: from human blood to social policy.* London, George Allen and Unwin.

Turner B. (1995) *Medical Power and Social Knowledge,* 2nd edn. London, Sage.

Wilkinson R. (1996) *Unhealthy Societies: the afflictions of inequality.* London, Routledge.

Williams A., Robins T. and Sibbald B. (1997) Cultural Differences between Medicine and Nursing and Implications for Primary Care. Summary Report, NPCRDC, University of Manchester.

Part One

Understanding the Social Context of Care

1

Society

Introduction

> Every human society is in the last resort men (and women) banded together in the face of death.

In Berger's (1967) words it is possible to catch a glimpse of the paradoxical nature of human life: we enter the world as individuals, experience illness alone and die alone. At the same time, we struggle against this tidal wave of nature. Collectively, we construct versions of birth, illness and death in order to make sense of our lives. For example, as Jordan (1983) observes, despite the universal physiological fact of birth, there are varying versions which reflect changing ideas and values characterising the societies which construct them. Birth in the USA has for decades been overwhelmingly conceived as a medical procedure. Birth in the Yucatan, Mexico, is understood as stressful but a normal part of family life. In Sweden, birth is experienced as an intensely fulfilling event and in Holland it is viewed as a natural process (Jordan 1983, p.34). It is interesting to note, as Jordan does in a more recent edition of her book *Birth in Four Cultures* (Jordan 1993, p.49), that the medicalized version of birth in the USA is changing (or at least diversifying) somewhat as the concept of 'family bonding' has taken hold. Similarly, as you will read in Chapter 9 of this volume, accounts of death are varied, complex and changing. Indeed, whether or not we are alive or dead becomes an issue largely insofar as we live in societies where the private and individual become public and political.

As nurses and others who are engaged in one way or another with the provision of health care, we are critically involved in the collective struggle to give meaning and purpose to life events such as birth, illness and death. For example, the medicalization of childbirth structures the relationship between a pregnant woman and a professional. The 'woman' is transformed into a 'patient' and this transformation has consequences. Whereas in another culture where childbirth is seen as natural drugs are precluded, drugs are likely to be given as a matter of course in a society where birth is overwhelmingly seen as a medical event (Jordan 1993, p.49). It is important for nurses, midwives and others who provide care for pregnant women (and for others in our care) to be aware of the social context within which we practise as individuals, and which we take so much for granted. Knowing that certain practices are bound by cultural expectations and values provides a basis from which to evaluate orthodox (and sometimes outmoded) practices. Thus it also provides a basis for action.

And so we turn to 'Society', a word we take for granted in everyday life, but nevertheless a word which sociologists have made the cornerstone of their discipline. In this first chapter we identify three important ways in which the word 'society' has been used by founding sociologists and contemporary sociologists in order to justify the discipline of sociology. First, we take a brief look at society 'as an idea'. As we shall discuss, it is an idea which has developed largely as a critique of individualism which, as we have indicated in the introduction to this book, is an idea associated with the enlightenment and which has left a legacy in the contemporary world. Second, we explore the dynamics of society. To do this we identify the concepts of culture, order and deviance, concepts which sociologists have defined and refined in order to determine and explain how society works. Third, we briefly consider some theories related to how society changes.

The purpose of our exploration of society in this first chapter is to begin to map the parameters of the context within which health care is practised and health issues are raised and debated. As with the remainder of the book, it is the authors' intention to bring to the readers' attention the relevance of sociology to making sense of health and illness. To this end, a number of texts are cited. We are particularly indebted to Martin and Sharrock (1995) whose illuminating account of the contribution of Marx, Weber and

Durkheim to sociology strongly informs our discussions. References also include sociological writings in the fields of culture, society, occupational sociology, medical sociology, power, sociologies of health and illness, including mental illness, deviance, and so on. As stated in the introduction and reiterated here, we do not wish to provide a comprehensive sociological account, in this case, of 'society'. Rather we hope to raise questions and to stimulate readers to explore in greater depth areas of discussion which may be of particular interest to them.

The idea of society

The idea of 'society' is central to sociology. Nearly all sociology textbooks refer to the word 'society' in one way or another. This is hardly surprising because, as most sociology textbooks infer, society is, at least at one level, about people. As Bauman (1990, p.8) explains, sociologists are interested in the ways that people 'are dependent on other people', 'live always (and cannot but live) in the company of, in communication with, in an exchange with, in competition with, and in cooperation with other human beings'.

However, society is conceived of as more than just the human beings who comprise a group at any one time (Babbie 1994, p.4). How is this possible? One way in which this is possible is to be found in the writings of sociologist Emile Durkheim which, as Hughes, Martin and Sharrock (1995, p.168) observe in their useful assessment of his work, show that the 'something more' than individuals consists primarily in shared patterns of behaviour or what would be called 'common' culture in contemporary sociology. That is to say the ideas, beliefs and values which give a group character and identity. Indeed Giddens (1990, p.32), another leading contemporary sociologist, sees society and culture as interdependent concepts.

A critique of individualism

Another way in which society can be conceived of as more than just human beings or, indeed, more than shared common culture is as a 'critique' or a political tool. We have already cited Hughes, Martin and Sharrock (1995, pp.7–10) as suggesting that:

> While it is dangerous to characterise a complex body of ideas in terms of a single theme, it is not too much of a distortion to describe the rise of sociology as part of a reaction against the individualism so prominently displayed in the thought of the enlightenment during the seventeenth and eighteenth centuries.
>
> (Hughes, Martin and Sharrock 1995, p.7).

These authors provide a useful summary of the rise of ideas about the 'reasoning individual', citing key theorists. For example, they cite Rene Descartes (1596–1650), famous for his statement about the human condition: 'I think therefore I am'. Thomas Hobbes (1588–1679) was another writer to take the idea of a reasoning individual as a basis for thinking about the human condition. He argued that civilization could only occur when aggressively competitive individuals realized the benefits to be gained from accepting the authority of a monarch.

Enlightenment thinkers laid the basis for the development of a set of ideas which supports the view that individuals' acts are governed by the rational calculation of self-interest. These ideas have influenced economics, politics and the discipline of psychology. Indeed as Hughes, Martin and Sharrock (1995, p.8) point out, these ideas have become part of the common sense of the modern western world that 'each of us is, or ought to be, a unique autonomous person, possessing free will and certain inalienable rights'.

Kingdom (1992), a political commentator, provides an example of how society as a critique of individualism has been applied in recent times. He takes Margaret Thatcher's proclamation that 'there is no such thing as society', a proclamation which, as he writes, captures the essence of a political mission which challenges ideas about community and collectivism, replacing them with an 'individualistic credo'. In contrast to the individualistic credo which asserts that people have selves independent of social formations, Kingdom argues (following many sociologists) that individuals are 'socially constructed; everyone is born into a social group which makes them what they are' (Kingdom 1992, p.6).

The idea that individuals are socially constructed or defined by society derives substantially from the writings of Durkheim. Hughes,

Martin and Sharrock (1995) discuss how Durkheim was concerned to bridge the gap between a 'freely acting' individual and a 'constraining', society. He bridged the gap by first rejecting the utilitarian view that individuals assess their actions in terms of whether or not they will lead to pleasure or the avoidance of pain. Although he acknowledged that people do concern themselves with these issues he believed they are also directed in their conduct by **moral** considerations of right and wrong. For example when we are hungry we look around for something to eat but we would stop short of eating each other. Second, he was concerned to bridge the gap between a 'freely acting' individual and a 'constraining' society by showing how a new member of a society learns and identifies with the moral order and is trained in the ways of the group he or she is entering; in short how individuals are 'socialized' into a group.

Durkheim developed his analysis to demonstrate the idea of society as a reality *sui generis* (in and of itself). He likened this entity to the human body. Just as a human body can be analysed as a system of interrelated parts, so too can society. However, Durkheim, it is suggested (Hughes, Martin and Sharrock 1995), used the body metaphor primarily to emphasize the importance of the science of society, a science concerned with 'social facts' and analogous to medicine insofar as Durkheim was concerned that sociologists should be able to diagnose society's ills and be able to suggest appropriate treatment. Importantly, Durkheim did not conceive of society in any simple way as a superior element in relation to individuals, rather that the two elements are interrelated (Hughes, Martin and Sharrock 1995, p.154).

In summary, the idea of society is important to sociology insofar as it is a reminder that explanations of everyday life should go beyond focusing on selves as independent of social formations. By social formations we mean groups and institutions through which individuals live together, cooperate, compete and enter into exchange with other people. These social formations include, for example, the family which we discuss in Chapter 2. They include methods of organizing professional concerns and interests which is a key focus of interest in later chapters.

The idea of society provides more than an explanation of how we engage with each other and the world around us. It also provides a basis for thinking about things differently from enlightenment ideas that have had and continue to have a tremendous impact on contemporary thought and action. Social theorists throughout the history of the discipline have shown how the latter is so. Founders of the discipline of sociology, for example Durkheim, Weber and Marx, have shown how ideas relating to society have the potential to provide alternative explanations to individualism in order to make sense of human everyday life. Contemporary sociologists (while often criticizing the founding sociologists) continue to do so. As we shall see, they may, however, emphasize aspects of society possibly unthought of by the founding sociologists in their analyses, such as ethnicity and gender.

The dynamics of society

In this section of the chapter we look in some detail at what constitutes 'the something more' than individuals referred to by Durkheim and re-visited by sociologists ever since in trying to determine and explain how society works. We turn first to the idea of culture without which, as Giddens (1990) suggests, it would be impossible to comprehend the idea of society.

Culture

Most anthropologists and sociologists would agree that culture, like society, is a shared supraindividual concept which as Gidden's points out has close connections with the idea of society. He writes that 'Culture' concerns the way of life of the members of a given society – their habits and customs, together with the material goods they produce (Giddens 1990, p.32).

The idea of culture as portrayed within this statement could be interpreted as simply the aggregate of independent traits. However, LeVine (1986, pp.67–77), an anthropologist, reminds us that that culture is a shared organization of ideas that includes the intellectual, moral and aesthetic standards prevalent in a community and the meanings of communicative actions. To summarize LeVine, an investigation of culture requires, therefore, an investigation of the general rules, concepts or assumptions that generate the particulars readily accessible to the investigator.

For example, LeVine (1986), commenting on culture in the context of his fieldwork experiences with the Gusii (the people he encountered in Kenya between 1946 and 1949), writes that when intense emotional experiences were reported by members of the Gusii, the form and content of the reports were standardized. He writes that these were 'apparently following a conventional script with a single set of symbols and meanings' (p.71). He continues:

> This conventional script . . . is what I would call a collective phenomenom, something supraindividual even though it informs individual experience.
>
> (LeVine 1986, p.71)

Moreover as LeVine documents, when he returned to the Gusii community in 1972 and met the new generation, the son of one of his old friends, a secondary school graduate, told him stories of life since LeVine's previous period of fieldwork some 17 years earlier. The stories, according to LeVine, were related in the same way as before. Levine comments:

> Here again I was confronted by the collective nature of a folk culture that had never been written down . . . read only by highly educated Gusii outside the the district) yet continued to shape personal experience. Such confrontations are common in ethnography and generate for many anthropologists the sense of culture as something shared, collective and supraindividual.
>
> (LeVine 1986, pp.71–72)

To give an example closer to home and to the interests of this book: an exploration of the particulars of the history of 'western' medicine suggests that ideas about health and illness are organized around the mind–body dichotomy, with distinctions drawn between psychiatry and medicine.

Cultural variation and diversity

For many anthropologists and sociologists, general rules, concepts or assumptions that generate the particulars of a culture vary from society to society. LeVine (1986) observes that using the 'western' categories of religion, medicine and psychology did not help him to understand the Gusii conceptual framework for explaining the situations of health and economic resources that affect individual well-being.

By contrast, Ahmad (1996) argues that there is a large degree of convergence between the health beliefs and behaviour of different ethnic groups even across countries and continents. He draws on the work of Kakar, a western-trained psychologist and psychoanalyst to make the point that there are points of convergence in the discourses of, on the one hand, demonological viewpoints and, on the other, experts on mental illness (pp.207–208), although there are, of course, differences. In making this point, Ahmad (1996, p.208) is well aware of the complexities of culture – that culture is political, changing, linked to economic and gender issues, and that there is cultural diversity within societies as well as between societies.

Diversity within cultures is illustrated by anthropologists (e.g.Okely 1996) and sociologists working in a number of areas. A sociological study which illustrates the complexity of culture is the by now classic study 'Learning to Labour' (Willis 1980). A feature of the study is that it focused on a group of school boys, a group which does not conform to certain accepted middle-class norms. Willis' school boys played truant and turned up for classes late. However, the boys did not breach all norms, for example they went into jobs approved by their families (Willis' study was carried out in the late 1970s). Their truancy resulted in poor educational attainment which in turn consigned them to working-class jobs which could be seen as a mechanism for maintaining the status quo.

The study is (amongst other things) a case illustration of different sets of norms and values. As in the study of US medical students by Becker *et al.* (1961), it is an example of student culture – a 'sub-culture', the 'underside' of society. A criticism of Willis' study is that it does not reflect the full complexity of cultural diversity. It does not take gender into account and the possibility that the homogeneously portrayed working-class values might be further differentiated if girls were taken into account within the study. For example, Okely (1996) shows how the middle-class public school experience in the 1950s was different for girls than the image portrayed which relied on the accounts of boys' schools.

The concept of culture is much debated within social anthropology and sociology. Culture is a word which takes on different meanings in different contexts, as will be elaborated in future chapters. However, it does provide a basis for looking at some of the ways in which society constitutes itself and the complexities of order, deviance and change in this process.

Order and 'deviance'

As Giddens (1990) writes, our activities would collapse into chaos if we did not stick to rules which define some kinds of behaviour as appropriate in given contexts (p.117). One of the contributors to this text recalls an instance from fieldwork (undertaken in a number of nursing settings) when a student nurse told her tutor that she was fed up with dealing with other people's problems, given the problems she herself was experiencing at home. Perhaps the words were said in a fit of pique or tiredness. Perhaps she was under real duress and at her wit's end. Whatever the understandable reasons for her outburst, the tutor pulled her up in no uncertain terms. The words the student had uttered reflected 'the wrong attitude' as the tutor stressed later. Perhaps a different tutor at a different time would have 'counselled' the student nurse rather than harangued her (as indeed was the case in another instance), but in both cases the (or rather 'a') public image of nursing is reinforced – that of 'professional', and the point remains that the action did not embody the norms appropriate to the situation. The student nurse's words were seen as 'deviant' in the particular situation.

It could be argued that at the moment the student nurse uttered the words that she was 'fed up', the boundary between nursing and non-nursing was threatened. This situation is reminiscent of Bauman's (1987, p.58) point about threatened boundaries between 'us' and 'them'. 'Us' refers to insider members of a particular group while 'them' refers to outsiders. Bauman makes the point that the boundary between insider and outsider can be threatened from the inside as well as the outside. Indeed he makes the point that many a political party, church or a nationalist or sectarian organization spends more much more time and energy fighting its own dissidents than its declared enemies. The student nurse is hardly a dissident insider. Is she an outsider? Could she be, to quote Bauman, 'someone not quite like us' (Bauman 1987, p.58)? At the moment of uttering the words 'I'm fed up' she could be conceived as '**student** nurse' and not 'nurse' – not yet a nurse and therefore not like the others present. If she were a nurse conceivably she would not have spoken that way.

Another factor which comes into play here is power. In the instance above, the tutor defined the action of the student nurse as inappropriate. She also had the power to make the label of 'inappropriate' stick. In the introduction to the 1994 edition of his classic book *The Established and the Outsiders*, Elias makes an important point about the role of power in establishing boundaries. He writes:

> Differentials in the degree of internal cohesion and communal control, can play a decisive part in the power ratio of one group in relation to that of another.
>
> (Elias 1994, p.xviii)

He continues with reference to Winston Parva a small suburban community:

> In that small community the power superiority of the old established group was to a large extent of this type. It was based on the high degree of cohesion of families who had known each other for two or three generations, in contrast to the newcomers who were strangers in relation not only to the old residents but also to each other. It was thanks to their greater potential for cohesion and its activation by social control that the old residents were able to reserve officers in local organisations such as council, church or club for people of their own kind, and firmly to exclude from them people who lived in the other part and who, as a group, lacked cohesion.
>
> (Elias 1994, p.xviii)

Elias then goes on to comment:

> Exclusion and stigmatisation of the outsiders by the established group were thus powerful weapons used by the latter to maintain their identity, to assert their superiority, keeping others firmly in their place.
>
> (Elias 1994, p.xviii)

Ideas relating to the maintaining of social boundaries and identities of individuals and groups are very much the province of a group of sociologists who have come to be known as 'interactionists'. Interactionists are concerned with understanding how people themselves interpret the social world. Unlike 'science' which draws on the positivist ideas of cause and effect and is preoccupied with uncovering general laws of society, interactionist sociologists have drawn on interpretive philosophies, including the work of Max Weber especially in relation to his elucidation of the concept of 'verstehen', which is understanding in the interpretive sense rather than in the sense that, for example, water boils when you heat it to a certain temperature.

Within this broad orientation, a specific area of interest exemplified by the work of Becker (1963), and Goffman (1959), is the exploration of the processes involved in constructing boundaries between 'conformity' and 'deviance'. The theory associated with this exploration is called 'Labelling theory'. Rather than seeing 'deviance' as caused by genetic inheritance or some personality defect, interactionists are interested in the processes by which people are identified or labelled as 'deviant' – the process of interaction between 'deviants' and 'non-deviants' (Giddens 1990, p.129).

The label 'deviant' is a negative label. On the whole it is used to describe the vulnerable and not the rich and famous. Ask yourself the question, is the Royal Family deviant? Even if your response was in the affirmative, it would be difficult in the present climate to make it stick. Keeping others firmly in their place depends on what Mary Douglas has called making the human-made order stick. Thus the term 'deviant' is applied by the **powerful** to describe the vulnerable.

The construction of illness as deviant behaviour

Within the sociology of health and illness in contemporary western society, there has been interest in how healthcare professionals construct illness as 'deviant' behaviour. In other words an interest in the processes by which boundaries are drawn between health and illness. Scambler's by now classic discussion of 'Deviance, labelling and stigma'(Scambler 1982, pp.184–192) provides a useful focus for considering the ways in which boundaries are constructed between health and illness by society in general, and by healthcare professionals in particular.

Scambler suggests that there are three main ways in which illness is constructed as deviant behaviour in the context of illness and health care. They are as follows: illness 'as' deviance, illness as affording special opportunities for deviant behaviour and, lastly, special or stigmatizing illnesses. Scambler (1982) points out that, 'some have contended that illness itself is a type of deviance because being ill is an unwelcome state'. Scambler quotes Freidson (1970), the author of *The Profession of Medicine*, who writes that 'human and therefore social evaluation of what is normal, proper or desirable is as inherent in the notion of illness as it is in notions of morality.' Illness, it is argued, represents a deviation from culturally established norms or standards of good health. Thus anyone acknowledged to be ill desires, and is the recipient of, treatment to correct his or her state of body or mind.

This argument raises questions about how fixed and obvious are the boundaries that are drawn between health and illness. In another classic work, Ivan Illich (1977) writes that aspects of life which could be easily viewed as 'normal' by some are medicalized by doctors, for example childbirth. Similarly, aspects of life which might be viewed as 'unfortunate' by some are medicalized by others, for example alcoholism.

Power is a factor which comes into play very strongly in a consideration of how boundaries are drawn between health and illness. In Illich's examples we can see how a professional group can construct an aspect of everyday life as 'a problem'. Indeed the professional group (e.g. doctors or counsellors or nurses) can make the resolution of the problem its province and its expertise.

This latter point is touched on by Scambler who argues that illness makes possible new and distinctive kinds of deviant behaviour. And he refers to Parsons (1952), who maintains that although a person who becomes acutely ill in countries like the USA is accorded certain rights, he or she at the same time acquires certain obligations, namely to be motivated to get well, and to seek help from, and cooperate with, medical experts. These rights and obligations, so his argument goes, are culturally entrenched. If on becoming ill people neglect their new obligations, they are likely to be regarded as malingerers or at least regarded as irresponsible or misinformed. Their behaviour deviates from what is both expected and required.

We can see how health professionals 'construct' a constituency or 'their patients'. An ill person is obliged to act like 'a patient', and to comply with health professionals. Power is again an issue. Foucault (whose contribution to sociology is further discussed in detail in Chapter 6) makes a number of observations about the instruments of power used by disciplines such as medicine. For example, examinations are instruments of power, and the labels 'healthy' and 'unhealthy' are labels which can be the result of examinations by a medical practitioner. Such examinations could result in the person/patient not being offered a mortgage or not being admitted to a particular profession or occupation.

Foucault also talks about 'normalizing judgement', which is a phrase he gives to the process whereby little punishments are given to draw attention to failure. These observations are part of the elucidation of an idea which has made Foucault famous – the idea of the surveillance of everyday life or hierarchical observation which put crudely means the ability of those at the top to keep an eye on the activities of those beneath them. Some may disagree with aspects of Foucault's analysis (e.g. Porter 1995) and others may disagree with those sociologists who have developed Foucault's ideas (e.g. 1977, 1980) in relation to healthcare workers, for example health visitors and others (Bloor and McIntosh 1990, May 1992). Many of us, however, will have experienced this kind of labelling, and we also may engage in it from time to time as healthcare professionals.

Scambler identifies a third way in which illness is constructed as deviant behaviour. He writes about specific illnesses which are regarded as deviant by lay populations: These, he says, are usually referred to as stigmatizing conditions. Thus people who are 'blind' (sic), victims of VD (he writes before the moral panic of AIDS), and mentally ill people have been ridiculed, shunned or isolated by non-sufferers. Here the issue of labelling is brought to the foreground of our attention. Labelling leads to stigma (Goffman 1973). When a patient is labelled as deviant (in the sense that she/he is given a stigmatizing official/professional label such as 'blind' or 'epileptic' or 'mentally ill'), then the label sticks. Becker wrote that a 'deviant' is one to whom the label has been successfully applied. Deviant behaviour is behaviour that people so label. Can we say that ill people are ill because we label them so? Scheff (1966) in his classic work *Being Mentally Ill: a sociological theory* writes that labelling was the single most important cause of mental illness in his study.

It is important to note here that there are those who disagree most strongly with this view. For example, within nursing, Cox (1989) sees this view as dangerous insofar as it turns attention away from pathology (e.g. biochemical/physiological problems as in schizophrenia). Cox's critique echoes W. Gove's (1970) by now famous critique of Scheff. Gove wrote a paper entitled 'Societal reaction as an explanation of mental illness – an evaluation' in which he points out that the majority of mentally ill people suffer from a mental disturbance **before** the label is applied. Gerhardt (1989) also reminds us of the importance of taking pathology seriously into account as people may be concerned about the physical symptoms of their disease. Nevertheless, we should take Scheff's criticisms seriously. It is important to acknowledge the view that labels have consequences. One consequence is that the stigmatizing label can come to dominate the perceptions that others have of a person, and how they treat that person. This is sometimes referred to as cultural stereotyping.

Scambler gives an example of cultural stereotyping, citing a piece of research carried out by R. Scott in 1969 called 'The Making of Blind Men', where Scott describes how, in his study, 'blind' people were differentiated from sighted people insofar as they are attributed with certain characteristics . . . helplessness, dependency, docility, melancholy, gravity of inner thought and aestheticism. Scambler then goes on to point out that however far-fetched the labels, it is difficult for 'blind' people to ignore how others expect them to behave. Scott lists the ways in which blind people react to this kind of cultural stereotyping which are as follows: by simply concurring, by cutting themselves off, by adopting a facade of compliance for expediency's sake, by making people pay for a 'performance', for example begging or by actively resisting (Scott 1969).

Healthcare professionals draw boundaries between health and illness in interesting and subtle ways. In doing so they reflect the prejudices of society. They also have power to make the labels of 'health' and 'illness' stick.

In this section we have looked at some of the ways in which society constitutes itself. We have also tried to convey the sense that this is a 'moral process' insofar as boundaries are constructed and justified according to ideas about what is normal and what is deviant behaviour. As suggested, this process is not obvious and straightforward and we have offered an account of some of the complexities involved. It is hoped that the references indicated in our discussion will provide a basis for a wider exploration of sociological literature in this respect. We next turn to a related area of discussion which is about society and change.

Change and society: theory and action

How one views and interprets change in society depends on where one is coming from both intellectually and politically. In his book *Thought and Change*, Gellner (1972, p.1) writes that 'societies exist in time' and that 'the way in which time and its horizons are conceived is generally connected with the way the society understands and justifies itself'. For example, if a society were to believe that it is unchanging in terms of excellence, time could be said to be 'morally neutral'. That is to say there is no conception of movement or change towards something 'better' or 'more excellent'. On the other hand if a society justifies itself as constantly improving and moving towards being 'better' then it is not morally neutral, of course.

The idea of progress

It is the latter justification or the idea of progress that characterizes the ways in which modern European society has been understood since the eighteenth century and almost until the present. Once again we return to the individualism displayed in the thought of the enlightenment of the seventeenth and eighteenth centuries and which influenced the classic economists, for example, Adam Smith who represented human nature as improving through acts governed by the rational calculation of self-interest. Similarly political theorists (e.g. Hobbes and Locke) saw the progress of the state and social order as agreement reached by reasoning human beings. To quote Gellner, 'the idea of progress was the great discovery of the eighteenth century' (1972, p.3).

The idea of progress remained. However, during the nineteenth century it became evident that ideas about how the benefits of the pursuit of self-interests would lead to improvement in the general welfare of all were not having the impact hoped for (Hughes, Martin and Sharrock 1995). Concerns about the growth of a massive working class living in conditions of poverty provoked a new enthusiasm for thinking about the nature of society. And so the individualism of the eighteenth century gave way in some respects to ideas about 'the social'. This is reflected in, for example, the emergence of proto-disciplines such as Saint Simon's 'social physiology', and Auguste Compte's 'social physics' which became 'sociology' (Harris 1968).

The association of the idea of progress with the social domain (as opposed to individualism) is illustrated by looking at the links between the work of Georg W.F. Hegel and the work of Karl Marx. Hegel saw the world as consisting of entities in dialectical relationship with their opposite, contradictory or negative ideas. As Harris writes in reference to Hegel's ideas:

> The tension between them reveals the evolutionary working of the world mind. Out of the "negation of the negation" there evolves a new entity or state of existence which in turn is meaningful only in relationship to its contradictory ingredients.
>
> (Harris 1968, p.67)

Hegel, as Hughes, Martin and Sharrock (1995) discuss, was interested in more than the workings of the human mind. Hegel was interested in the maturation of 'collective' resources. He wrote about the 'spirit of a time' or the 'spirit of a nation'. These are as suggested by Hughes, Martin and Sharrock (1995) similar to what we might call 'culture' today. However, while drawing to some extent on Hegel's ideas of contradiction, conflict and transformation, Marx was concerned with 'real people' rather than the 'spirit of a time'.

For Marx, society was the outcome of the struggles of real people or classes of people pursuing their interests. Marx was writing at a time when theorists were trying to make sense of changes from 'agrarian society' to 'industrial society'. The focus was on explaining the processes of industrialization. Marx believed that the contradictory interests of the capitalists (those who owned the means of producing material goods – the means being the factories, tools and other resources) and the workers (those whose labours were bought) would result in growing working-class consciousness and resistance to the orthodoxy. Indeed Engels in the preface to the English edition of 'Capital' (Marx 1978, p.112) writes 'the theories of Marx, even at this moment, exercise a powerful influence upon the socialist movement which is spreading in the ranks of "cultured" people no less than in those of the working class'.

Consensus and conflict theories

'Progress' in the sense of moving towards something better was seen by Marx as related to class and, importantly, class struggle and conflict. Here Marx diverges from the idea held by his near contemporaries, predominantly Durkheim, that the natural state of society is one of dynamic equilibrium. From this latter perspective 'progress' in society was associated with the 'healthy' expansion of the legal and administrative apparatus of sociality and of an appropriate set of moral and ethical rules (Harris 1968). This crude summary of the views put forward by Durkheim and his contemporaries is given the shorthand term 'consensus theory' in many sociological textbooks.

The term 'consensus theory' tends to overlook important aspects of Durkheim's contribution to sociology. As Hughes, Martin and Sharrock (1995) point out, the association of Durkheim with consensus theory or functionalism, as is it sometimes undertood, overlooks certain radical elements in Durkheim's thought. They write of the importance he attached to the cause of reform and stress how:

> Indeed, his whole conception of sociology as a diagnostic tool was predicated on a conception that much in the society of his day needed changing. However, this could be achieved not by returning to some putative Golden Age, as conservative social theorists often tended to argue, but by serious scientific inquiry into the working of the complex social order to lay the basis for the rational reform of society.
>
> (Hughes, Martin and Sharrock 1995, p.206)

Here we catch glimpses of Durkheim's critique of crude individualism: individuals need to feel a sense of solidarity with others. Without family and other ties – to, for example, religious or political groups – men and women may find life has no meaning such that 'everything becomes a pretext to rid ourselves of it' (Durkheim 1951, p.213). Durkheim's analysis of sucicide as an act of anomie rather than an unpredictable human act underlines his firm commitment to the idea that it is society that defines a particular individual's wants, rather than the reverse. Readers may wish to consult Durkheim in the original for the detail of his analysis of suicide or Hughes, Martin and Sharrock's excellent evaluation of his work (1995; see Chapter 4). Here we would want to underline the point that Durkheim was convinced that social integration is necessary for an individual to play a constructive role in society and in order to develop his/her own capabilities.

In contrast to consensus theory, conflict theory emphasized conflict of interests in society. For example, Marx held that there is a conflict of interests between capital and labour. Hughes, Martin and Sharrock write:

> In the process of realising profits, capitalists must resist the claims of workers for higher wages, for the higher the wage bill the less the surplus value that will be created, and the lower the eventual profit. To this end, capitalists will seek to maintain a "reserve army of labour", as Marx put it, of unemployed people whose availability for work will act to restrict wage demands. (p.73)

The idea that wealth alone determines power was strongly criticized by the sociologist Max Weber (1864–1920). Weber was interested in explaining social action in terms of the meanings people attribute to their actions rather than in terms of social structures such as preset rules which constrain behaviour. He was interested in the creativity demonstrated by people in responding to their environment, rather than accepting that people respond to an economic stimulus. Weber saw competing forces at work in society, such as political parties, professional groups and trade unions (Cuff, Sharrock and Francis 1990; Giddens 1990).

Other theorists have criticized the Marxist preoccupation with class struggle to the exclusion of other struggles. Although, as Harris (1968, p.236) points out, 'the Marxian strategy was remarkably free of the endemic racism of the nineteenth century', race was not a priority. Neither was gender, and in Chapter 2 we shall explore critiques not only of the idea of progress but also of the founding sociological analysts' general neglect of gender and race in their analyses of the family and health and illness, whether consensus or conflict.

Summary

In this first chapter, we have explored an idea which has become a hallmark of sociological analysis. We have looked in some detail at the dynamics of society – how boundaries are constructed, justified and maintained in the face of potential transgressions. We began to explore how boundaries are constructed between 'health' and 'illness', and how the constructions vary depending on situational factors such as who is constructing them and the specifics of a situation. These processes and the associated issue of power are revisited in later chapters, particularly in relation to lay and professional views of ill-health.

As already discussed in the Introduction to the book, one way in which sociology can be understood is as a critique of individualism. Within this broad understanding of sociology the idea of society provides a rallying point. In this sense, society is an idea which has had, and continues to have, political significance. How one views and interprets 'society' – indeed whether or not one accepts it as a reality – depends on where one is coming from both intellectually and politically. Readers will note that the political significance of ideas and institutions is a recurring feature of discussion throughout the remaining chapters.

References

Ahmad W.I.U. (1996) The trouble with culture, in Kelleher D. and Hillier S. (eds) *Researching Cultural Differences in Health*. London, Routledge.

Babbie E.R. (1994) *What is Society: reflections on freedom, order and change*. Thousand Oaks, Pine Forge Press.

Bauman Z.(1990) *Thinking Sociologically*. Oxford, Basil Blackwell.

Becker H. (1963) *Outsiders*. New York, Free Press.

Becker H., Geer B., Hughes E. and Strauss A. (1961) *Boys in White: student culture in medical school*. Chicago, University of Chicago Press.

Berger P. (1967) *The Sacred Canopy: elements of a sociological theory of religion*. New York, Doubleday.

Bloor M. and McIntosh J. (1990) Surveillance and concealment: a comparison of techniques of client resistance in therapeutic communities and health visiting, in Cunningham-Burley S. and McKeganey N. (eds) *Readings in Medical Sociology*. London, Tavistock/Routledge, pp.159–181.

Cox C. (1989) *Sociology: an introduction for nurses, midwives and health visitors*. London, Butterworths.

Cuff E.C., Sharrock W.W. and Francis D.W. (1990) *Perspectives in Sociology*. London, Unwin Hyman.

Durkheim E. (1951) *Suicide: a study in sociology*. London, Routledge.

Elias N. (1994) *The Established and the Outsiders*. London, Sage.

Engels F. (1978) Preface to the English edition, in *Capital: a critique of political economy*, Volume 1. Harmondsworth, Penguin in association with New Left Review.

Foucault M. (1977) *Discipline and Punishment*. London, Allen Lane.

Foucault M. (1980) The eye of power, in Gordon C. (ed) *Power/Knowledge*. Brighton, Harvester Press.

Freidson E. (1970) *The Profession of Medicine*. New York, Dodd Mead.

Gellner E. (1972) *Thought and Change*. London, Weidenfeld and Nicholson.

Gerhardt U. (1989) *Ideas about Illness*. London, Macmillan.

Giddens A. (1990) *Sociology*. Oxford, Polity Press.

Goffman E. (1959) *The Presentation of Self in Everyday Life*. London, Pelican Books.

Goffman E. (1973) *Stigma*. London, Penguin.

Gove W. (1970) Societal reaction as an explanation of mental illness – an evaluation. *American Sociological Review* 35, 873–884.

Harris M. (1968) *The Rise of Anthropological Theory.* New York, Columbia University Press.

Hughes J., Martin P. and Sharrock W.W. (1995) *Understanding Classical Sociology.* London, Sage.

Illich I. (1977) *The Limits to Medicine.* Harmondsworth, Penguin.

Jordan B. (1983) *Birth in Four Cultures: a cross cultural investigation of childbirth in Yucatan, Holland, Sweden and the United States.* Montreal, Eden Press Women's Publications.

Jordan B. (1993) *Birth in Four Cultures: a cross cultural investigation of childbirth in Yucatan, Holland, Sweden and the United States* (revised and expanded by Davis-Floyd R.) Prospect Heights, Illinois, Waveland Press.

Kingdom J. (1992) *No Such Thing as Society? Individualism and community.* Buckingham, Open University Press.

LeVine R.A. (1986) Properties of culture: an ethnographic view in Shweder R.A. and LeVine R.A. (eds) *Culture Theory: essays on mind, self and emotion.* Cambridge, Cambridge University Press.

Marx K. (1978) *Capital: a critique of political economy.* Harmondsworth, Penguin in association with New Left Review.

May C. (1992) Individual care? Power and subjectivity in therapeutic relationships. *Sociology* 26(4), 589–602.

Okley J. (1996) *Own or Other Culture.* London, Routledge.

Parsons T. (1952) *The Social System.* London, Tavistock.

Porter S. (1995) *Nursing's Relationship with Medicine.* Aldershot, Avebury.

Scambler G. (1982) Deviance, labelling and stigma in Patrick D.L. and Scambler P. (eds) *Sociology as Applied to Medicine.* London, Baillière Tindall, pp.184–192.

Scheff T. (1964) The social reaction to deviance: ascriptive elements in the psychiatric screeing of mental patients in a midwestern state. *Social Problems* 2, 401–413.

Scheff T. (1966) *Being Mentally Ill: a sociological theory.* New York, Weidenfeld and Nicholson.

Scott R. (1969) *The Making of Blind Men.* New York, Russell Sage Foundation.

Willis P. (1980) *Learning to Labour: how working class kids get working class jobs.* London, Gower Press.

2

'The family'

Introduction

Sociologists generally agree that 'the family' is a most important institution for sociological investigation. Nearly all sociology textbooks, including textbooks addressing health and illness, explore ideas about 'the family'. While there is agreement amongst sociologists about the importance of understanding and explaining 'the family', there has been considerable debate about its role and purpose in contemporary society. Gittens (1987) writes, 'some argue that the family is the foundation of society, indeed, of civilisation itself. Others maintain it is the source of most of our problems and unhappiness' (Gittens 1987, p.1). In this second chapter we aim to give an indication of the breadth and divergence of sociological accounts of 'the family', 'family' or 'families', bearing in mind Morgan's (1996, p.14) observation that family practices have a key place in the analysis of a complex and fluid society.

We then turn to a problem which appears to preoccupy contemporary sociologists and non-sociologists alike. The problem is related to the question: is the family in decline in contemporary UK society? It is not simply that sociologists feel compelled to answer the question yes or no. Rather it is that in exploring the question we learn more about the paradoxical nature of family life. We encounter what at first glance may appear to be contradictory issues around what constitutes a family: on the one hand, sociologists describe a diversity of family patterns and changing relationships; on the other hand, we note the tenacity of 'the family' as an ideal which has become entrenched in contemporary culture and politics. Finally, we ask the question: what do sociologists have to say about the relationship between family life and health in contemporary society? Here, we want to consider the family as a context for promoting or threatening health. We conceive of health in its widest sense.

Throughout the chapter we argue that our discussions provide us not only with an understanding of 'the family' and its relationship to health, but also with a sense of what sociology is about. To reiterate the point we make in both the 'Introduction' to the book and in Chapter 1, 'Society', how institutions are interpreted depends on where one is coming from politically as well as intellectually. Sociologists are not morally neutral commentators on society and its institutions but have a view of how things ought to be which infuses their work. As Morgan (1985) writes in his excellent analysis of 'the family': 'family theorising does not take place in a social and economic vacuum. Some theoretical approaches derive directly or indirectly from actual practice . . . while some therapeutic and political practices have . . . been influenced by theoretical themes' (Morgan 1985, p.266). It is precisely through a process of noting the political as well as the intellectual features of sociological arguments that we can evaluate the contribution of sociology to understanding the family and its relationship to health in contemporary society.

Sociological accounts of the family

Sociologists are not united in their views and explanations about the family and how it has developed as an institution in contemporary society. In their diverse interpretations of major family theorists, sociology textbooks provide us with a range of analyses of what is paradoxically one of the most taken-for-granted institutions in history.

Consensus accounts

A predominant way of providing an analysis of the family in many of the textbooks which introduce students to sociology and the sociology of health is by first noting the contributions of consensus theorists including Talcott Parsons, and Robert Murdock who defined the family as a social group characterized by common residence, economic cooperation and reproduction. From a consensus perspective the family includes adults of both sexes, at least two of whom maintain a socially approved sexual relationship, and one or more children, own or adopted, of the sexually cohabiting adults' (Gittens 1987, p.60). The unit may be 'extended' to include adults from more than one generation or it may be 'nuclear' (consisting of parent[s] and child[ren]). These, by now, classic sociologists are often referred to by contemporary sociologists as 'functionalists' whose conception of societies was as systems of interrelated and interdependent parts (Elliott 1991).

Functionalists have emphasized how the family is a global institution with specific functions (as noted above – common residence, economic cooperation, reproduction and sexuality) essential to a society's survival (Gittens 1987, p.60). Overall, from a functionalist or consensus perspective the family is a healthy institution which provides an infrastructure of support and care based on ideas of commitment and duty and which, thus, contributes to the health of a society. Some anthropologists have stressed that kin relations within the family constitute a 'special' category of social relationships which carries the obligation to offer assistance and to share resources when necessary. For example, as Finch and Mason (1993, p.8) note, Fortes writing in 1969 comments that 'kinship is binding; it creates inescapable moral claims and obligations'. As we discuss later in both this chapter and in Chapter 3, this view of kinship persists in contemporary society and, arguably, has been used to justify major health policy initiatives such as care in the community.

As you would expect, this somewhat optimistic consensus or functionalist perspective has its critics. The critics are introduced in textbooks as 'conflict theorists' (e.g. Jones 1994). The latter category is sometimes referred to as 'critical perspectives' (Morgan 1985) and this category is further subdivided to convey the scope of possible critiques. We focus here on two major contributions to challenging functionalist views of the family, namely Marxist theory and feminism, although we would stress that neither category is exclusive nor homogeneous.

Marxist theory

Morgan asks the question, 'in what respects would conventional sociology of the family be held wanting in the light of a Marxist critique?' (Morgan 1985, p.212). Morgan goes on to highlight how this might be so in general terms which he writes might also apply to other strands of critical thought (by which we take him to mean feminism, psychoanalytical theory, the Frankfurt School). A main point of the critique, according to Morgan, is that to talk of 'the family' in conventional social scientific terms (we understand Morgan to include the functionalist perspective in his discussion of conventional sociology) is to understand the family as 'naturalistic, static and individualistic' (Morgan 1985, p.212). He writes, 'a universal family is also a family without history. Conventional sociology, further, has a tendency towards methodological individualism, treating the individual as the basic unit of analysis' (Morgan 1985, p.213). He explains that the tendency to individualism is expressed by 'more or less universal psychological or biological needs whose site of origin may be said to be "the individual" and at the level of actual sociological practice by the use of questionnaires and other individually centred research techniques'(Morgan 1985, p.213).

Morgan's words reflect the sociological concern to offer a critique of 'individualism' which we discussed in the introduction to the book and in Chapter 1, where we noted how early social theorists' use of the term society could be understood as a critique of the individualism of enlightenment thinking. However, Morgan's words also draw to our attention how difficult it is to maintain a sociological critique of individualism when, as he notes, individualistically based research techniques are employed to explore what is perhaps otherwise seen as an 'holistic' institution or an institution (to follow Durkheim) which is 'something more' than individuals.

By contrast, Morgan (1985) suggests that within a Marxist framework of analysis there is at least a commitment to viewing the family as a product of history and to exploring the economic relationship between the family and society. Central to understanding the relationship between the family and society in traditional Marxist theory was an analysis of the institution of primogeniture, which is the passing on of family wealth from father to first-born male offspring. Primogeniture, as Morgan points out, provides a clear link between the family and the societal institution of private property. He comments on this:

The family becomes an institution within which there is a whole nexus of inter-related interests and processes: the familial control over property within a generation and its passing on between generations; the concern to produce legitimate male offspring; patriarchal control over women and children; the desire to establish profitable (or at least non loss-making) alliances and so forth. Thus too we have links and continuities between the "natural" family of married couples and legitimate offspring and a class society; the family becomes a central institution in the reproduction of class inequalities.

(Morgan 1985, p.214)

The Marxist emphasis on the family as a focus for economic relationships rather than relationships of a moral nature where people act out of a sense of duty and obligation has influenced sociologists and anthropologists, for example, Worsley (1956) and Bloch (1973) as Finch and Mason discuss (1993, p.8). Similarly, the Marxist analysis of the family as a central institution in the reproduction of class inequalities has influenced sociologists, including those writing about class as a factor in unequal provision of, access to and uptake of, health in contemporary Britain as we shall discuss in Chapter 3. However, Morgan is not suggesting that Marxist theory provides the 'best' sociological account of the family. This is far from the case. Morgan's work on the family (1975, 1985) gives a critical account of a range of critical perspectives (Marxist, feminist, psychoanalytical, the Frankfurt School). In his critique of Marxist theory Morgan points out that while marxists have been successful in identifying and analysing the 'external' economic relationships, they are less successful, 'as feminists have noted', in exploring the dynamics of economic activity and control within the household where gender differentiation plays a significant role' (Morgan 1985, p.215).

This is a point that Elliott (1991) picks up on in her analysis of the family and she notes that in mainstream Marxist accounts of the family, 'man' is the reference point of analyses which focus on class divisions within society 'and see the family as structured by capitalist imperatives' (Elliot 1991, pp.12–13). This is the main point of contention in feminist accounts of the family to which we turn next.

Feminist accounts

Feminist sociologists and feminists working in related disciplines have made a major contribution to understanding contemporary family life. They have been critics of both functionalism and orthodox conflict perspectives including Marxist theory (Morgan 1985; Cuff, Sharrock and Francis 1990; Giddens 1990; Elliot 1991). Broadly, feminist writings about the family take a conflict perspective. However, whereas Marxists emphasize class divisions within the overall framework of capitalism, feminists take as their starting point gender divisions – conflicts and differences of interests between men and women – and they take 'patriarchy' as their frame of reference (Elliot 1991, p.13). The key theme of feminist critiques of both functionalism and orthodox conflict theorists of the family is that they either ignore women or do not take them seriously in their analyses. This point is elaborated by Stanley and Wise (1983, 1993), who write:

> The most simple and in many ways the most powerful criticism made of theory and practice within the social sciences is that, by and large, they omit or distort the practice of women.
>
> (Stanley and Wise 1993, p.27)

Stanley and Wise draw on a number of feminist scholars to support their contention including Oakley (1974) who, as they point out, examines possible explanations for why the practice of women is distorted – why there is sexism in sociology, noting that at the origins of sociology lie the 'sexist interests' of its 'founding **fathers**' interests which persist throughout the recent history of sociology, reflecting a view of reality which is informed by an 'ideology of gender' which leads people to construe the world in sexually stereotyped ways (Oakley as cited by Stanley and Wise 1993, p.27). Founding fathers include functionalist sociologists who, as Frieden wrote, advocated a strict division of roles between males and females in the domestic sphere (Stanley and Wise 1993, p.28) to Marxists who relegated 'the woman question' to the margins of their interest and concentrated on the male breadwinner and 'the family wage' in discussions of the family in relation to the public economic sphere (Morgan 1985, p.220).

Even the term 'family' has male connotations as Gittens (1987, p.35) reminds us. She writes that implicit in the concept of the western family is the notion of male, specifically paternal ('paterfamilias'), dominance over others. Thus, Gittens (1987, p.35) writes: 'by definition the family has been an unequal institution premised on paternal authority and power'. This pervasive unequal distribution of power within the family has been largely ignored in conventional discussions about sex roles such as 'mother' and 'father' in the family. So that any changes in roles have been viewed optimistically to indicate increasing democratization within the family, as reflected in the by now classic work by Young and Wilmott (1973) in which they proposed that relationships between men and women in families are more equal than they used to be, this assertion is based on records of the sharing of domestic work between spouses.

Unequal distribution of power within the family has of course been recognized by Marxists as we have seen in the discussion of primogeniture; and it was Frederick Engels in his book *The Origin of the Family, Private Property and the State* (Engels 1978) who in 1884 commented that within the family the woman was 'the proletariat' while the man was 'the bourgeois' which, as Morgan notes, emphasized the presence of sexual antagonism within the family. However, Morgan continues:

> at the same time the metaphorical use of the class terms does suggest that sexual antagonism was regarded as being of somewhat secondary importance and, to a large extent, dependent apon economic class struggles.
>
> (Morgan 1985, p.215)

Feminists by contrast have insisted on looking beyond sex role analyses and seek to seriously investigate how the family not only serves to perpetuate class but also gender inequalities. They do this by bringing to the forefront of sociological attention the deep-rooted inequalities which are part of the everyday experiences of most women, that is the fact or the threat of male violence in the home or on the street (Morgan 1985, p.241), as well as the constraints of domesticity (Oakley 1974), giving birth (Oakley 1980), financial subordination within marriage (Graham 1987) and the stresses and strains of domestic responsibility which some have argued result in women's ill-health (Graham 1984). We take up this latter point later on in this chapter.

The main organizing factor in feminist critiques of both functionalism and Marxist theories of the family is the use of the term 'patriarchy'. The term 'patriarchy' has been used to organize questions of power between women and men around these and other facts of oppression. However, its precise definition and use has been debated and contested within feminism. For example, one definition of patriarchy is: 'The universal oppression of women and younger men by older men' (Millett 1970). Eisenstein (1979) argues that patriarchy and capitalism should be examined as interdependent systems, but this according to Morgan (1985) and Elliott (1991) is problematical insofar as it does not take into account the political dimension.

Elliott suggests the following and somewhat general definition of patriarchy which is: 'the ways in which power relations between men and women, and men and children, are exercised and defined' (Elliot 1991, p.36). The main point is to show that patriarchy is relevant to understanding families. Indeed as Gittens (1987) observes, patriarchy permeates and influences society at all levels: political, economic, ideological and familial. She writes that the essence of patriarchy:

> lies in a concept of a social order premised on a male, but particularly paternal, authority which by definition presupposes the dependence and service of children and other "inferiors".
>
> (Gittens 1987, p58)

Feminists aim to challenge the idea of social order premised on the male. This means challenging functionalist assumptions about the family which reinforce the orthodox, patriarchal order and Marxist imperatives to subordinate the study of gender differences to class differences. Thus feminists study the family from a women's perspective. In doing this, as Morgan notes, feminists have offered a profound critique of the main assumptions that have guided sociological research and theorizing. In the following discussion we look at an example of how feminist work on the family, as indeed in other areas, involves a radical critique of sociology in respect of theorizing and methods, drawing on the work of Dorothy Smith (1988).

Smith (1988) asks in relation to the family, what effect does the 'odd' role of mother which as she notes is 'lacking in authority and overburdened with responsibility for outcomes over which she has little control' have on women? What are the implications of this role for family relations? (Smith 1988, p22). Smith goes on to suggest that questions like these require an approach which preserves the presence of subjects of research. She then demonstrates how such research might be designed and she includes in her discussion the example of how research might be designed from her own experience as 'a single parent'. She comments on how this piece of research ('qualitative' research called ethnography involving participant-observation) would be a part of a complex of different women's experiences (a number of ethnographies) which, when placed together, provide an analysis of the organization and relations of 'women at work as mothers in relation to children's schooling' (Smith 1988, p.202).

Smith's work not only presents another perspective on the social world including the family but also a different way of theorizing and understanding social life and institutions insofar as she begins to dismantle boundaries constructed between, on the one hand, professional or academic knowledge and, on the other hand, lay knowledge (Smith 1988; see Chapters 4 and 5). At the heart of this approach lies a concern with making visible what is so often taken for granted in sociological analyses of the family among other institutions, that is questions about what counts as knowledge. Feminist critiques of the family may vary but they are united in the recognition that what counts as knowledge about the family is largely male based, mediated by male interests; and that such knowledge should be reviewed in the light of what is actually experienced.

In this section of Chapter 2 we have tried to give a sense of the variety of ways in which sociologists try to understand the family. We give only a glimpse of the diversity of accounts available to us and urge readers to consult where possible classic authors such as Parsons, Marx and Engels in respect of the family, as well as contemporary authors who have reviewed in depth writings on the family (e.g. Elliott 1991; Finch 1989; Gittens 1987; Morgan 1975, 1982, 1985, 1996). We have tried to begin to give a sense of some of the key debates in family theorizing, namely: is 'the family' universal or is it possible, as Gittens suggests, 'to begin to see the historical and cultural specificity of what is really meant when reference is made to "the family"'(Gittens 1987, p.72). Does the family have a distinctive moral character or are relationships within the family essentially the same as other relationships, such as those concerned with material and economic interests?

These questions reflect some of the debates between classical functionalist and Marxist theorists and they have been revisited and explored by feminists and other contemporary sociologists as we shall see as we continue to explore the paradoxical nature of the family.

The paradox of the family

As suggested earlier an exploration of issues around the question 'is the family in decline in contemporary society?' provides us with insights into the paradoxical nature of the family. In our discussion of the paradox of the family we draw on themes that appear to be common to sociological accounts despite the heterogeneity of the discipline. They are about what constitutes a family. On the one hand writers comment on the diversity of family patterns and changing relationships. At the same time, and to reiterate the point we made earlier, there is recognition of the tenacity of 'the family' as an ideal which has become entrenched in contemporary culture and politics.

Diversity and change

We return to Murdock's definition of the family as a social group characterized globally by the following functions: common residence, economic cooperation and reproduction. Gittens (1987) suggests that we look critically at each of these functions in turn in order to challenge the general functionalist assumption that the family is universal and to show instead that it is an institution characterized by diversity of forms.

Gittens (1987) argues that in terms of common residence, anthropologists have shown how different groups organize themselves in households which do not equate with 'family household'. For example, Mead (1971) showed how Samoan children chose the houshold where they wanted to reside, and often changed their residence again later. Gittens observes that in contemporary UK society where partners have jobs some distance away from one another they maintain a second household where one of them lives during the week (Gittens 1987, p.61).

As far as economic cooperation is concerned, Gittens points out that because all resources are finite and some are scarce we cannot assume that they will be distributed cooperatively. Graham (1987) in her study about being poor and coping with lone motherhood supports Gitten's contention when she explains how lone-parent mothers in the study recalled difficulties in accessing money for housekeeping from their past wage-earning partners when they were living with them. Graham explains that a common theme with the mothers in her study was that although financial resources were very tight they felt less poor being single than with a wage-earning partner. They felt, and indeed had, more control over the limited resources to which they had access.

Gittens discusses the inadequacy of the functionalists' equation of family with reproduction, arguing that functionalists tend to conflate reproduction with sexuality, the assumption being that their definition of sexuality is heterosexuality and that this should be a defining characteristsic of families, notwithstanding anthropological evidence to the contrary which suggests that not all marriages (understood as socially recognized customs of mating and parenthood) are heterosexual. Drawing on Edholm (1982), she gives the example of the Nuer where older women may marry younger women. She also relates how the Nuer practise a custom known as ghost marriage where when an unmarried or childless man dies, a relation then marries a woman 'to his name' and the resulting children of this union are then regarded as the dead man's children and bear his name.

The main point of Gitten's argument is that functionalist accounts of the family cannot take account of the diversity of arrangements for the organization of co-residence, economic relations, sexuality and reproduction. She suggests that kinship is a more useful term than 'the family'. She writes that it is:

> concerned with the ways in which mating is socially organised and regulated, the ways in which parentage is assigned, attributed and recognised, descent is traced, relatives are classified, rights are transferred across generations and groups are formed.
>
> (Edholm 1982, p.166)

As Gittens points out this definition stresses that kinship is a social construction and while some anthropologists are sceptical about how far one can leave biology out of kinship (Gellner 1987), kinship as a concept offers a framework for accounting for the diversity of meanings which may attach themselves to concepts like family obligations and family responsibilities. This is what Finch and Mason (1993) show in their book *Negotiating Family Responsibilities*. They are concerned to explore how far taken-for-granted assumptions about what a family member may or may not do for another family member (which so often directs policy makers' expectations of family self-help) are reflected in ways in which kin relationships operate in practice. They write:

> it is not enough simply to assume that the family as a social institution is ready, willing and able to shoulder the burden of supporting its members who cannot fully care for themselves, either practically or financially.   (p.10)

Here of course Finch and Mason are challenging functionalist conceptions of inherent moral rules associated with genealogical positions. What they go on to argue is that while they disagree with the idea of fixed rules in relation to family responsibilities, they found in their study that people did have a flexible conception of 'guidelines' . . . 'in the sense of considerations which it is appropriate to take into account in working out whether to offer assistance to a relative' (p.9). In contrast to Marxist theorists, they argue that in following the guidelines which structure negotiations about who should do what for whom . . . the people in their study did not simply engage in assessing the material value of what they were giving (and receiving), but also engaged in constructing and reconstructing themselves as moral beings (p.170). In showing how this is so they very usefully contribute to bridging 'either/or' dichotomies between functionalist preoccupations with moral rules and Marxists' preoccupation with how material considerations govern reciprocity within the family.

In the discussion so far we glimpse the diversity and fluidity of 'family' forms. We have mentioned partners who live in different households, lone parents, same-sex partnerships. Earlier in the chapter, we mention that the nuclear family was thought by some to be a response to the demands of industrial society (Giddens 1990, p.391). In other words the nuclear family has superseded the extended family (often associated with agrarian society in recent British history). This view has been contested by historians (Laslett) and sociologists alike (see Morgan 1985; see Chapter 8 for a full account), and Morgan suggests that the 'before' and 'after' industrialization model of understanding changes in family structure is rather limiting (1985, p.161). Finch and Mason (1993) suggest that the extended family still exists in contemporary Britain. They write:

> At the simplest level, our study updates the work of researchers who looked at family and kinship in Britain in the 1950s and 1960s [Young and Willmott 1957, Bell 1968, Rosser and Harris 1968, Firth Hubert and Forge 1970]. They concluded that, despite widespread beliefs to the contrary, the extended family was alive and well, and had a tangible reality in most people's lives. We are saying that, thirty years later, it still does.
>
> (Finch and Mason 1993, p.163)

Some theorists argue that growing recognition of diversity and fluidity of family forms is reflected in the terminology sociologists use (Berger and Berger 1983, pp. 59–65). For example writers may use the word 'families' rather than 'the family'. We should also note that not only is there diversity of form but also that a single family changes composition and form over time with children being born, leaving home, the death of a spouse and so on. The changing composition of a family over time is further complicated by cohabitation, separation and divorce, lone parenthood and step-parenthood.

At this point we could return to the question we raise earlier: is the family in decline in contemporary Britain? On the one hand, it could be argued that the diversity of family forms is leading to a situation where the family is in decline in contemporary UK society. Indeed recent statistics from the 1991 Census would appear to support this argument (Central Statistical Office 1994). For instance, more than a quarter of households in 1991 consisted of one person living alone – almost double the proportion in 1961. For every two marriages in the UK in 1991 there was one divorce. Over the last decade the proportion of births outside marriage has doubled to almost one in every three births in 1992 (Central Statistical Office 1994, p.33).

However, despite recognition of diversity and change, theorists argue that whenever the terms 'the family' or 'families' are used there remains ambiguity and contradiction. For example, Elliot points out that 'change in terminology does not solve the definitional problem for it raises the question: "what is it that is varying but is regarded as familial?"' (Elliot 1991, p.6). We explore this problem next.

The family as an ideal

Elliot's question takes us to the heart of the paradox of the family. Characterized by diversity, the family 'as an ideal' seems to be important in contemporary UK society. People in general see the family as the cornerstone of civilization, and UK politicions across all parties have called for the return to so-called family values. Gittens (1987) suggests that the ideology of 'the family' in contemporary society is such that it affects our lives. She writes that the family is seen as the 'bulwark' of our culture and notes how 'ideals of family relationships have become enshrined in our legal, social, religious and economic systems which in turn, reinforce the ideology and penalise or ostracise those who transgress it' (Gittens 1987, pp.71–72). We all know of people in the public eye who by 'threatening' their marriages through infidelity are made the subject of media 'sleaze' exposures. And at a more general and everyday level people's attitudes to family forms (e.g. reconstituted families where remarriage takes place after divorce; lone parents) which do not emulate the ideal suggest that these family forms do not seem quite as correct as mainstream nuclear families. For example, lone-parent families have been constructed by politicians as 'problem' families.

As well as ostracizing people who 'transgress the ideals of family relationships', there is a tendency by society to react 'positively' to tackle 'marital problems' and to save threatened families through counselling and other means. For example, when divorce is imminent people attempt to prevent it, where possible. There is an attempt to work through the problems which threaten to disrupt the family. Family members may intervene, and counselling is available through general practitioners and organizations such as 'Relate'. Morgan writes that this tendency reflects a process which he calls the 'medicalisation of marriage'. He writes:

> To treat a class of marital problems called 'marital problems' is to recognise or endorse the centrality of a particular definition of marriage within society as a whole. To refer to marital problems is to enter into some kind of tacit agreement or negotiated understanding between patient/client and professional/therapist about the importance and centrality of this relationship.
>
> (Morgan 1985, p.35)

Morgan draws on Foucault to make the point that problems of marriage and family matters have entered the domain of medical influence. Indeed what constitutes a problem is constructed by the medical profession (it was once constructed by the church). We can then draw on Foucault to suggest that marriage and the family have become further areas of everyday life for medical surveillance. The main point is that Morgan's analysis underlines how the ideal of 'the family' is perpetuated and managed within society. As feminist writers (e.g. Barrett and McItosh 1982) argue the family is safe from decline precisely because it serves the purpose of an essentially capitalist and patriarchal society.

Thus we are left with the paradox that, despite diversity and change, 'the family' exists as a persistent ideal in contemporary Britain. It is an ideal which informs health policy as well as well as everyday health practices. There is also another aspect to idealizing family life as the proper and moral context for perpetuating the health and happiness of women, men and children. That is to say if the family is seen as unquestionably 'good', the dark side of family life including the misuse of power resulting in violence and the abuse of family members remains hidden. Feminists have on the whole been very critical of the taken-for-granted view that the family is a 'good' institution, and it is mainly to the work of contemporary feminist sociologists that we now turn to comment, critically, on the relationship between family and health.

The relationship between family and health

In her, by now, classic book *Women, Health and the Family*, Graham (1984) writes that 'for most of us it is families which met our health needs in childhood: for warmth and shelter, for love and comfort'. She continues:

> Families, too, serve as our first and most significant health teachers. In adulthood, most people create new families (often more than once). to support them "in sickness and in health". In old age, it is our family, again, who cares most and does most for us.
>
> (Graham 1984, p.17)

A complex relationship

Graham's words encapsulate the complexity of the relationship between family and health. From one perspective we have an image of family life characterized by caring and giving. It is an image which may or may not make sense in the light of our own experience of growing up, and certainly it is an image with which we are familiar as nurses, healthcare workers and others who tend to promote the notion of family-centred care and health.

From another perspective, we note a degree of irony in the notion that most people create new families to support them 'in sickness and in health'. The words suggest a degree of self-interest which may not at first glance sit easily with notions of caring and giving. In this respect Graham's words suggest that reciprocity is an issue to be considered seriously in any exploration of the relationship between family and health. The role of reciprocity in establishing relationships is a topic which has engaged sociologists and others since Marcel Mauss wrote his famous work *The Gift,* in which he explores the significance of the giving and taking of gifts, and the variations on this process. Earlier we noted how Finch and Mason (1993) consider reciprocity in their analysis of family responsibilities. To reiterate, Finch and Mason are concerned to explore how far assumptions about what a family member may or may not do for another family member are actually reflected in ways in which kin relationships operate in practice. They point out how, in doing things for other family members, people engage in constructing and reconstructing themselves as moral beings (p.170). Radley (1994) in his discussion of reciprocity in relation to 'the sick role' (following Parsons), uses the notion of 'moral credit'. He explains how moral credit refers to the process by which a person who gives care is thereby owed a debt. He writes by way of example:

> A husband might complain of "feeling a cold coming on" and suggests to his wife that he might stay at home "to prevent it getting worse". Both of them realise that his symptoms hardly merit his staying away from work, but the wife may use this opportunity of offering the "gift" of the sick role to her husband, saying that if he stays at home she will look after him. In this case it is the wife to whom a debt is owed, through her gift of care and consideration.
>
> (Radley 1994, p.79–80)

For whatever reasons, the family is a key locus for health work. Although as Graham (1984) points out 'when we look at family life, it is sometimes difficult to see that a large part of what parents do is work for health' (p.150). She makes the important point that certain terms commonly used to describe what a family does obliterate the health dimension. For example, the term socialization is used to describe the process by which children are reared to accept the ideas that give a group identity. However, as she reminds us it is a term which fails to convey the fact that parents ensure the survival as well as the socialization of their children. She writes that while we emphasize the importance of mothers in shaping the minds of children, we may be blind to their role in building and repairing bodies (p.150).

Graham lists the various kinds of health work performed by families (mainly mothers) as the provision of a materially-secure environment involving warm clean accommodation, purchasing of food and the provision of a diet to meet nutritional needs. She refers to the labour-intensive work created by illness in the home. Health teaching is another area of work involving the setting of standards of diet and hygiene. Mediating with outsiders, for example with doctors and health visitors, about the care of children (pp.150–151) is another aspect of the health work undertaken by parents.

A further aspect of health work undertaken by parents and other family members and one which precedes (or may take the place of medical intervention as noted by Cunningham Burley (1990, p.85) refering to Hannay (1979, 1980) and Spencer (1984)), 'mediating with outsiders', is discussed by Radley (1994) as the 'lay referral system', whereby members of families (as well as friends in some cases) act as advisers to family members who are anxious or uncertain about a symptom such as a lump in the breast or hearing loss. Radley discusses how uncertainty about a symptom may result in what looks like the activation of a referral network whereby a number of people are consulted before the person with the symptom actually consults a doctor. However, as Radley emphasizes, the network is not there waiting to be activated. Rather it is more a matter that the network comes into being in the course of discussions with the person with the symptom or worry and those who are advising them. We take Radley's point here to echo, at least in part, Finch and Mason's (1993) contention that there are no fixed rules governing family obligations. Rather, caring work whatever its nature is accomplished through complex processes of negotiation. Obligations are acknowledged, however resources are utilized depending on the particulars of a situation.

Negotiation is not evident in all family relationships in respect of all aspects of family health. For example, Graham refers to study by Dobash and Dobash (1982) who record that 'arguments' (as opposed to negotiation) about food provided the trigger for violence between partners. With children Graham reports how 'treats' (as opposed to negotiation) play a crucial role in the management of children in public places (Graham 1984, p.134).

A key point in Graham's analysis is that the responsibilities of health work can often be in conflict with one another. For example, in trying to provide a nutritional diet for children the parents' nutritional needs may be compromised if resources are scarce (Graham 1984, pp.168–169). Thus Graham points to another aspect of health work often taken for granted, which is the coping with conflict aspect of meeting family health needs.

Structural vis individualistic explanations of family health status

Graham focuses on conflicts throughout her analysis of families and health. For although she recognizes that individual expressions of warmth, love and care are components of family life, she is well aware of problems associated with the health work of families. She goes on to discuss in detail how warmth, shelter, love and comfort are not evenly distributed across all families in contemporary Britain. Nor are they evenly distributed within families, and where they exist they do so often at the cost of the main carer's health (Graham 1984, *passim*).

On the theme of class in relation to health inequalities, Gittens (1987) observes that despite the great poverty surveys of the late nineteenth century drawing attention to the relationship between poverty and poor health, there has been a tendency to see illness and death, particularly the high rate of infant mortality, in terms of working-class ignorance of 'proper family life', domestic routine and careful child rearing (p.144). More recently the Black Report (1980) and associated publications (Townsend and Davidson 1982; Townsend, Davidson and Whitehead 1988), aspects of which are considered in Chapter 3 ('Community'), have established links between social class and health inequalities. However, despite evidence of the contribution of structural factors to health status, the tendency to focus on individual families as responsible for their health persists.

Radley (drawing on Donovan 1984) make this point in relation to the prevalence of lung cancer and heart disease in social class categories IV and V. He notes how behaviours or beliefs of these groups are targeted for change. Working-class people are advised to give up smoking without any exploration of the socioeconomic situation or of the role of smoking in the everyday lives of the people concerned. Pearson (1986) also makes a similar point in relation to the prevalence of rickets among Asian babies. She points out that a campaign to irradicate rickets commenced in the 1950s and by the end of the 1970s rickets was identified by the DHSS as an Asian problem. She continues:

> For reasons which are still debated and unclear, the DHSS decided not to fortify chapati flour in the way that margerine and cereals had been fortified for the white community twenty years before. Instead a change in Asian diet to those foods which had been fortified years before was encouraged, and more Asian women were extolled to expose themselves and their children to sunlight [DHSS 1980].
>
> (Pearson 1986, p.48–49)

As Pearson notes how the relationship between vitamin D deficiency and poverty was overlooked, as was Asian women's anxiety about going out into the sunshine for fear of racist attacks. Asian people were perceived to have an unhealthy diet because of their ignorance about nutrition (Pearson 1986, p.49). Here, as in Chapter 1, we have an example of the individualistic credo (Kingdom 1992) which asserts that people have selves independent of social formations.

On the theme of gender in relation to health inequalities, Barrett and McIntosh (1982) in their book *The Anti-Social Family* write that the family is antisocial because it exploits women. There is an assumption in family life that the woman will do the caring work and where care is lacking, women – wives and mothers – are blamed and indeed blame themselves. Graham takes up this point, arguing that the everyday family health work (which is in the main done by wives and mothers) and the anxieties this can provoke produce ill-health where resources are scarce and support is virtually non-existent. She points out that the assumption that women are primary carers, together with individualistic ideas about self-help in contemporary British society have led to the ill-health of women, particularly working-class women.

Graham's, by now, classic argument (1984) centres initially on three sets of statistics:

1. Statistics which suggest that women consult GPs more often than men (p.56).
2. Statistics which suggest that women rather than men are more likely to report periods of chronic ill-health (p.56).
3. Statistics which show that more women than men are classified as having neurotic and depressive disorders (p.78).

Graham suggests that the first set of statistics relates to the health work women do for other family members. This includes taking ill children to the doctor and well children for immunizations; pregnancy; contraception; and consulting physicians on behalf of and with elderly dependent family members. In relation to the second and third sets of statistics, listed above, she suggests that the biomedical response would appear to see the women as 'neurotic'. Whereas men presenting with similar symptoms will be diagnosed as 'overworked' and suffering from 'burnout', women will be diagnosed as mentally ill or 'neurotic'. Graham writes that far from being neurotic, women suffer from burnout because of the health work they do for other family members. Graham was writing in the middle 1980s . . . the question we have to ask ourselves is this, how far has the situation changed in the last decade?

Summary

Our aim in this chapter has been to give readers a sense of the complexity of a largely taken-for-granted institution in our everyday lives and one which is tied quite intimately to our health and well-being. Part of the complexity portrayed is a function of the efforts of sociologists to understand 'the family'. During the course of the chapter we move from orthodox accounts which take a consensus view to critical accounts of the family, primarily Marxist and feminist accounts. Throughout the chapter, the critique of individualism identified in the introduction to the book informs the various sociological analyses of the family and family health issues. The theme of inequality is similarly present. In the following chapter both themes are revisited in the context of an exploration of the idea of community.

References

Barrett M. and McIntosh M. (1982) *The Anti-Social Family*. London, Pluto Press.

Berger B. and Berger P.L. (1983) *The War over the Family*. London, Hutchinson.

Bloch M. (1973) The long term and the short term: the economics and political significance of the morality of kinship, in Goody J. (ed.) *The Character of Kinship*. Cambridge, Cambridge University Press.

Central Statistical Office (1994) *Social trends,* volume 24. London, HMSO.

Cuff E., Sharrock W.W. and Francis D. (1990) *Perspectives in Sociology.* London, Unwin Hyman.

Cunningham-Burley S. (1990) Mothers' beliefs and perceptions of their children's illnesses, in Cunningham-Burley S. and Mekegarey N. (eds) *Readings in Medical Sociology*. London, Tavistock/Routledge.

Delphy C. and Leonard D. (1992) *Familiar Exploitation: a new analysis of marriage in contemporary western societies*. Oxford, Polity Press.

Dobash R. and Dobash R. (1982) The violent event, in Whitelegg *et al.* (eds) *The Changing Experience of Women*. Oxford, Martin Robertson in association with the Open University.

Donovan J.L. (1984) Ethnicity and health: a research review. *Social Science and Medicine* 19, 633–670.

Edholm F. (1982) The unnatural family, in Whitelegg *et al.* (eds) *The Changing Experience of Women*. Oxford, Martin Robertson in association with the Open University.

Eisenstein Z.R. (ed.) (1979) *Capitalist Patriarchy and the Case for Socialist Feminism*. New York, Monthly Review Press.

Elliott F.R. (1991) *The Family: change or continuity?* London, Macmillan.

Engels F. (1978) *The Origin of the Family, Private Property and the State* (following the English translation published by The International Publishers, New York 1942). Peking, Foreign Languages Press.

Finch J. (1986) *Research and Policy*. Brighton, Harvester Press.

Finch J. (1989) *Family Obligations and Social Change*. Cambridge, Polity Press.

Finch J. and Mason J. (1993) *Negotiating Family Responsibilities*. London, Routledge.

Frieden B. (1963) *The Feminine Mystique*. Harmondsworth, Penguin.

Gellner E. (1987) *The Concept of Kinship and Other Essays*. Oxford, Basil Blackwell.

Giddens A. (1990) *Sociology*. Oxford, Polity Press.

Gittens D. (1987) *The Family in Question*. London, Routledge.

Graham H. (1984) *Women, Health and the Family*. Brighton, Harvester Press.

Graham H. (1987) Being poor: perceptions and coping strategies of lone mothers, in Brannen J. and Wilson G. (eds) *Give and Take in Families*. London, George, Allen and Unwin, pp. 56–74.

Hannay D.R. (1979) *The Symptom Iceberg: a study of community health*. London, Routledge and Kegan Paul.

Jones L. (1994) *The Social Context of Health and Health Work*. London, Macmillan.

Kingdom J. (1992) *No Such Thing as Society? Individualism and Community*. Buckingham, Open University Press.

Laslett P. (1971) *The World We Have Lost*, 2nd edn. London, Methuen.

Mauss M. (1954) *The Gift*. London Cohen and West.

Mead M. (1971) *Male and Female*. Harmondsworth, Penguin.

Millett K. (1960) *Sexual Politics*. New York, Doubleday.

Morgan D.H.J. (1975) *Social Theory and the Family*. London, Routledge and Kegan Paul.

Morgan D.H.J. (1982) *Berger and Kellner's Construction of the Family*. Occasional Paper No. 7. University of Manchester, Department of Sociology.

Morgan D.H.J. (1985) *The Family: politics and social theory.* London, Routledge and Kegan Paul.

Morgan D.H.J. (1996) *Family Connections: an introduction to family studies.* Cambridge, Polity Press.

Oakley A. (1974) *The Sociology of Housework.* London, Martin Robertson.

Oakley A. (1976) *Housewife.* Oxford, Martin Robertson.

Oakley A. (1980) *Women Confined: towards a sociology of childbirth.* Oxford, Martin Robertson.

Pearson M. (1986) Racist notions of ethnicity and culture, in Rodmell S. and Watt A. (eds) *The Politics of Health Education.* London, Routledge and Kegan Paul.

Radley A. (1994) *Making Sense of Illness: the social psychology of health and disease.* London, Sage.

Smith D. (1988) *The Everyday World as Problematic: a feminist sociology.* Milton Keynes, Open University Press.

Spencer N.J. (1984) Parents' recognition of the ill child, in MacFarlane J. (ed.) *Progress in Child Health.* London, Churchill, Livingstone.

Stanley L. and Wise S. (1983) *Breaking Out: Feminist Ontology and Epistemology.* London, Routledge.

Stanley L. and Wise S. (1993) *Breaking Out Again: feminist ontology and epistemology.* London, Routledge.

Townsend P. and Davidson N. (1982) *Inequalities in Health.* Harmondsworth, Penguin.

Townsend P., Davidson N. and Whitehead M. (1988) *Inequalities in Health: the Black report. The health divide.* Harmondsworth, Penguin.

Worsley P. (1956) The kinship system of the tallensi: a re-evaluation. *Journal of the Royal Anthropological Institute.* 86, 37–75.

Young M. and Wilmott P.L. (1973) *The Symmetrical Family.* Harmondsworth, Penguin.

3

Community

Introduction

As with 'society' and 'family', 'community' is an idea which appears
to defy easy definition. It is an idea which has been debated and
examined from a number of perspectives, and which has been used
by sociologists to convey the complexity and diversity of social
relationships. Some of the ways in which community has been
conceptualized include: as 'a locality' which is geographically located,
as 'a network of relationships' or as 'a type of relationship built on
caring and sharing' (Jootun and McGhee 1996, p.40). In this chapter,
we shall be looking at sociological analyses of the idea of
'community' and their implications for health and health care,
especially for nursing. The following questions will guide our
discussions: What can sociologists tell us about the idea of
community? How far can sociological perspectives on community
help us to understand health and healthcare issues? Throughout we
will consider the implications of our discussions in this chapter for
nursing.

What can sociologists tell us about the idea of
community?

A brief review of sociological literature suggests that sociologists are
clearly interested in the idea of community, and they reflect on its use
in contemporary society. Raymond Williams in his book 'Keywords'
(1984) writes that the word community never seems to be used

unfavourably. Sometimes the word is used to convey gentleness, sharing and caring (as in community care) and at other times it is used to convey positive action (as in community action). In both cases it is used positively. Williams' main point is that 'community' is generally taken for granted by society as something which is positive. You may want to ask yourself the question: how often has this 'positive' image of community been used by politicians to achieve changes in healthcare policy?

Leaving that question aside for the moment, we might ask at this point in the discussion the question: do sociologists, themselves, hold a 'positive' understanding of the idea of community? Joel Richman, in his useful text *Medicine and Health*, writes that sociologists, like the rest of society, have tended to idealize the notion of community either implicitly or explicitly in their various writings (Richman 1987). He cites Nisbet (1967), who suggests that a major preoccupation in the nineteenth century was for the 'loss' of community, a preoccupation engendered by the impact of two revolutions – the French and the industrial revolutions. Richardson writes how the fabric of the old order – a sense of community embedded in traditionalism – was eroded by the 'rise of new classes, by secular philosophies of legitimacy, by mass movement from the land, and by the new capitalist mode of production stressing individual competitiveness and success' (Richman 1987, p.187).

According to Richman, Tonnies gave the clearest formulation of the problem of loss of community in his book *Gemeinschaft and Gesellschaft* published in 1887. Tonnies spelt out the characteristics of gemeinschaft (community) which he attributed to pre-industrial society and gesellschaft (association) which he attributed to the new order emerging in the wake of industrialization (Richman 1987, p.188). Gemeinschaft was based on kinship, neighbourhood and friendship while gesellschaft was based on impersonality, change and decisions based on rational calculation. With industrialization and associated technological and social changes, gemeinschaft gave way to gesellschaft and its loss was felt or at least theorized by social theorists.

In the 1950s, sociologists Young and Willmott researched urban communities and family life and kinship in London's East End. In their classic work *Family and Kinship in East London* (Young and Willmott 1957), they argued for a closely knit working-class community, echoing the positive idea of gemeinschaft where kinship, neighbourhood and friendship underpinned working-class life. Sociologists who draw on gemeinschaft to illuminate working-class life have been criticised for their romantic view of working-class community by a number of sociologists. Cornwell's work, culminating in her book *Hard-Earned Lives*, provides a useful critique in which she distinguishes between, on the one hand, the public accounts of kinship, friendship and concern for others and, on the other hand, private accounts given by people which demonstrate a concern with self and one's own interests (Cornwell 1986). While we may want to challenge Cornwell's rather too clear-cut distinction between public and private, she shows how there are differences between the accounts of different groups; for example, men and women, young and old. In short, Cornwell argues for an understanding of community as heterogeneous and contradictory in character rather than the straightforwardly romantic version.

Drawing on Wolff's book *The Sociology of G. Simmel* (1950), Richman suggests that another famous early sociologist, Simmel, followed Tonnies in lamenting the loss of wholeness and community. However, Weinstein and Weinstein (1993, p.76) suggest that, unlike his contemporaries, Simmel's work is characterized by a 'decided lack of nostalgia'. Rather, Simmel has been described as a sociologist who struggled and engaged with the tensions of modern life, a 'pathfinder' who, it could be argued, laid the basis along with other social theorists such as Durkheim for the reappropriation of the lost spirit of community in the new social order.

Manifestations of engaging with the tensions of everyday life are varied and could be said to include Schumacher's (1960) idea of 'small is beautiful', which has influenced not only city planners, but also political thinkers of both the right and left (Richman 1987, p.191), resulting in the shift of care from 'institution' to 'community', in particular care for the mentally ill and the elderly. However, ideas about community and 'holistic care' are qualified by ideas related to the market such as efficiency and cost-effectiveness. And whether or not community is beautiful depends on one's experience of it. From one perspective, 'decarceration' (following Scull, 1983), that is to say putting those who were once in institutions into the community, is justified by economic theories which assert that the process of decarceration drives down costs of labour given the view that the workhouses and asylums did not pay for themselves. From another perspective, it has meant being left with the burden – the practical and emotional labour – of caring for dependent relatives without adequate resources, as feminist sociologists have discussed (e.g. Finch and Groves 1983).

Clearly, sociologists interpret the idea of community in different ways. Some have idealized community, but never simply and unproblematically. And then there are those who look very critically at the idea that community is all things positive. A, by now, classic example of social commentary on community which portrays a strongly negative view is Michael Ignatief's book *The Needs of Strangers* (1985). Ignatief reverses the notion that community is all things positive and asylums are dehumanizing and should be closed down. He reminds us that asylums were once places of respite while the community was a 'wilderness'. Over the years, he argues, the meaning of the words changed, possibly as a consequence of the 1830 poor laws when people without work were forced into harsh workhouses and other intitutions leaving us with a negative view of asylum and a positive view of community. Indeed, this is the view reflected in studies which include Goffman's (1968) work in closed psychiatric institutions in the USA, and which fuelled the anti-institutional mood of the 1960s and onwards, and which had some influence on public thinking and government policy for moving patients into the community. Although, as we have suggested, ideas about a caring, compassionate community constitute but one justification for policy change, another justification is the economic one about efficiency and cost-effectiveness – but at whose expense?

How far can sociological perspectives on community help us to understand health and healthcare issues?

Ignatief dramatically draws attention to the sociological message that the meaning of the word community can differ depending on one's experience of it. This message is important insofar as it highlights two important and overlapping imperatives. First, **we cannot afford to take for granted** even the concepts which are pivotal to our profession and practice such as 'community nursing', 'community care' and so on. What, from one perspective, may look warm and caring could, from another perspective, appear harsh and exploitative. As nurses, it is important to retain a critical stance. Given the often strongly positive connotations of the word 'community' this can be quite difficult.

Second, our critical stance should take account of the range and diversity of experiences. Whether community is conceptualized as 'a locality', geographically located or 'a network of relationships' where everyone knows everyone else or 'a type of relationship built on caring and sharing', it is never homogeneous. Above all, what is interesting about community is the paradox that while community infers commonality there is always the possibility of difference. This is a sociological point, which is to say that sociologists have made it their business to identify and explore differences in everyday life. There are a number of ways of showing this in relation to health, and indeed we will be exploring in later chapters differences of point of view (e.g. lay and professional views of ill-health) and differences of interest. As well, and as previously discussed in the Introduction to the book, difference is an idea that is available to, and used by, both those who uphold individualism and by those who challenge it. In short, there is a political dimension to how difference is explored. In this chapter, we look at how sociologists have investigated difference 'as inequality' in the context of a discussion of access to health and health care, thus highlighting inequalities which exist in a community in this respect.

Inequalities in health in the community

Why do people's experiences of access to health (as well as other resources and opportunities) differ? This question is central to sociologists' efforts to understand inequalities in society. And for nurses, as well as for other healthcare workers, this question is pressing as in the care we give we may be privileging some groups of people above others, not because they have been consciously prioritized as a group but because of taken-for-granted assumptions, prejudices and preferences. As Freund and McGuire (1995, p.201) suggest, because 'ideology (which they earlier describe as a system of ideas that explains and legitimizes the actions and interests of a specific sector) shapes people's expectations and what they consider to be evidence, it often produces evidence that confirms those expectations'. The authors continue, 'If, for example, I expect old people to be befuddled, my observations of them are likely to confirm my expectation'. As nurses, we may not even bother to engage people in serious discussion of issues which concern them if we think of them in this way. As health visitors, for example, if we expect young, working class, lone mothers to be ignorant of 'careful childrearing', then our words may help to construct barriers against effective communication. Similarly if, as healthcare workers, we believe Asian women to be ignorant about 'good nutrition', then we will interpret any health problems in the light of that belief, precluding, perhaps, a full understanding of the complexities of the situation, and the particular difficulties faced by a specific woman.

As we have suggested in Chapters 1 and 2, some people and groups of people are more powerful than others, and they would have the power to make labels like 'befuddled' or 'ignorant' stick, thus perpetuating stereotypical images which prejudice the health of individuals and groups on the basis of their class, race, gender, age and geographical location. In the following discussion we take class, gender, race and age, and we look at these variables in relation to health, also noting their relationship with each other in order to try and account for the complex ways in which inequality manifests itself.

Class

Class is a concept that we tend to take for granted, although how it should be conceptualized has long been the subject of debate amongst sociologists. Both Marx and Weber saw class as a key to understanding industrial capitalist society. As previously noted, for Marx, class was an economic entity. A class referred to a group of people characterized by their common relationship to a mode of production. For Marx a two-class society existed composed of the capitalists (bourgeoisie) and the workers (proletariat). Capitalist technology and work relationships forced the workers to sell their labour to capitalists, the dominant class. Any profits over and above what was needed to cover the costs of production (including the workers' wages) went into the hands of the capitalists. This led capitalists to drive down wages and, subsequently, led the working class to act collectively to strengthen their bargaining power.

Weber's understanding of class was more widely conceived to include the possession of specialist skills, status, prestige and 'party', by which he meant the power exercised by various groups including religious groups and political parties. For Weber, class was more than economic. Specialist training and expert knowledge gave certain groups of workers (accountants, doctors, lawyers) positions of power in relation to the capitalist class – the latter being those who owned the means of production (e.g. the factory owners).

Class and health

It is interesting to note how Marx's and Weber's ideas have influenced discussions of the relationship between class and health. Take, for example, the Registrar General's five-fold classification of class where occupation is a key indicator of class. The classification presented echoes Weber's ideas about class in some respects. The classification was first produced in 1911 and has since usefully demonstrated inequalities in relation to 'a wide range of social and economic attributes' . . . It has justified its existence as a variable which highlights important differences that are related to the social position of the individual (Central Statistical Office 1975).

However, the Registrar General's classification has its limitations. In pointing these out, Townsend, Davidson and Whitehead (1990, p.40) suggest that the classification tends to give attention to 'general standing' or 'prestige' of occupations rather than to 'material' differences. They suggest that when using the Registrar General's classification, the term 'occupational class' should be used as opposed to 'social class'.

Townsend, Davidson and Whitehead (1990) also hint at the complexities involved in understanding inequalities in health and, while they focus on class, they do acknowledge that an understanding of health inequalities must go beyond a class analysis. For example, they point to difficulties in using a married man's occupation rather than a married woman's occupation as an indicator of class inequality, especially when analysing the health of children. Arber (1991) is an example of a sociologist who has demonstrated that it may be misleading to rely on social class groupings, based on a male head of the family's occupation, in relation to infant and perinatal mortality.

At the beginning of Chapter 1, we noted how we are concerned to show how there is a link between, on the one hand, theories put forward to explain terms like society, family and community and, on the other hand, practical politics. Inequalities in relation to community is a case in point. In the introduction to their book 'Inequalities in Health', Townsend, Davidson and Whitehead (1990) write that 'inequalities in health are of concern to the whole nation and represent one of the biggest challenges to the conduct of government policy' (p.1). The book brings together in one volume two key reports: 'The Black Report' and 'The Health Divide'. The former was published, eventually, in 1980 after prior dismissal by the Secretary of State in the then new Conservative administration. It lays out the marked class differences in mortality and morbidity rates, especially in relation to chronic illness in the UK. The publication of 'The Health Divide' a decade later confirmed the main conclusion of the former report (Townsend, Davidson and Whitehead 1990, p.6) and added weight to the argument that we live in a society where class inequalities in health continue to exist.

Indeed, some 5 years later a *British Medical Journal* editorial (Anon 1994) points out how despite the British government's signature on a World Health Organization target to reduce inequalities in health by 25% by the year 2000, 'the country has gone rapidly in the opposite direction'. In the same volume, Wilkinson (1994, p.1113) writes:

> The 1980s were marked by an unprecedented widening of income differences and a growth of relative poverty in Britain . . . .. Widening material differences during the decade were accompanied by widening differences in mortality and by a substantial rise in mortality among men ages 15–44 in the poorer electoral wards.

And Phillimore, Beattie and Townsend (1994, pp.1125–1128) present findings which show that mortality differentials widened between the most affluent and deprived fifths of wards in all age categories under 75 years in their study to identify relative and absolute changes in mortality in the northern region of England between 1981 and 1991.

The study, 'Death in Britain' (Dorling 1997) arrives at similar conclusions, stating that 'areas in Britain which are the poorest deciles in terms of health are also the poorest in terms of affluence on a number of indicators' (residents in house with no car, children in households with no work and adults under 65 with a long-term illness).

Such social scientific analyses constitute an important critique of the idea that inequality is functionally necessary in society. The latter idea holds that differences and variation are unavoidable. Jones (1994) in her critique of this idea suggests that from this latter perspective, illness is not seen as a consequence of material inequalities, but rather as the result of 'conscious or unconscious retreat from social roles, as deviance' (Jones 1994, p.195). The work of Black, Whitehead and Townsend and others which stresses the links between material inequality and health and illness acts as a counter to the increasingly prevailing idea about personal responsibility for health, where an individual's behaviour is seen as the major factor in their health status.

The latter idea has fuelled health promotion strategies in recent decades; for example, the Health Education Authority's 'Look after Yourselves' campaign of the 1980s. A positive campaign in some respects, a major criticism is that it appeared to ignore the point that access to material resources make a difference to health and quality of life. This is nowhere more evident than in some of the posters displayed in the 1980s. For example, in the 1980s a health education poster depicting a pregnant woman smoking was accompanied by the slogan that smoking would damage the baby's health. In at least one ironic instance, the poster was placed on a hording along a busy polluted inner city road, passing through a deprived area along which business people and academics drove to and from work and home in leafy suburbs.

The problem with the 'Look after Yourselves' campaign was its assumption that changing behaviour holds the key to health. While undoubtedly there is some merit in this approach, taken alone it ignores the complexity of health status. It is important for nurses and other healthcare professionals to consider, first, how far their work follows models which are based on the presumption that a change in behaviour equals an unproblematical improvement in the health status of their patients and clients. Second, it is important to consider how this presumption leads to the belief that people who do not heed health promotion dictates are not deserving of care. Examples of trusts who have supported health professionals in their decision not to treat patients who smoke are a case in point.

While from one perspective the fostering of personal responsibility for health may appear to be a sensible strategy, from another perspective it just does not make sense where there are no resources in place such that people are in a position to make decisions about their lifestyles and health. Hilary Graham (1984) writing over a decade ago reminds us how for some the so-called decision to choose between, for example, healthy and non-healthy food is not an option. Rather compromises are made based on money available and other priorities in the daily lives of people with very few material resources.

Sociologists and other social scientists who explore the links between class, material deprivation and health have made an enormous contribution towards understanding inequalities. However, one could argue that while their contributions to understanding health inequalities are important, a limitation of some studies which explore links between material deprivation and health (e.g. Phillimore *et al.* 1994 and Wilkinson 1994) is that they assume a rather unilinear approach to understanding health status and experience. They do so because they focus on men and they focus on men within a particular age group, that is to say they ignore those above the age of 75, an increasingly growing sector of the population.

In the following discussion, we note some of the interlinking factors which draw our attention to further complexities involved in understanding health status and experience.

Connecting class, age and gender

The importance of connecting class with gender and age is a point made by Arber and Ginn in their paper 'Gender and inequalities in health in later life' (1993). Arber and Ginn write:

> It is ironic that research on inequalities in health largely neglects those age groups with the greatest ill-health and highest use of health resources, namely elderly people. (p.33)

They make the important point that 'the elderly' is not a homogeneous group, and they make a case for taking elderly women as well as men seriously into account, drawing on Bearon (1989):

> Elderly women report health as their most frequently mentioned source of dissatisfaction and their dominant concern in considering the future.
>
> (Arber and Ginn 1993, p.33)

The authors also underline how it is not advisable to treat the category 'elderly women' as undifferentiated, although they reject the tendency to differentiate on the basis of chronological age 'commonplace in the social gerontological literature . . .' suggesting that:

> Such distinctions are predicated on the assumption that chronological age is the fundamental determinant of health and other aspects of well-being in later life. (p.33)

In contrast, they point out that it may be the case, for example, that 'working-class women in their late 60s have an equivalent health status, and thus need, for health and informal care, to middle-class women in their late 70s or early 80s'. (pp.33–34).

Arber and Ginn take a political economy perspective in making their main case, which is that class and material advantages such as owning your own home, having access to a car and having a relatively high income are all associated with better health. In their edited collection of papers, *Connecting Gender and Ageing* (Arber and Ginn 1995), they emphasize the need to establish a theoretical connection, commenting that sociologists have tended to 'add on gender' to age relations rather than integrating gender as a fundamental relationship of social organization (Arber and Ginn 1995, p.2). They write:

> This failure to connect gender and age theoretically seems odd in view of the fact that most older people are women, but may reflect the origin of second wave

feminism, which began in a movement of mainly young women, a generational revolt. The lack of sociological research on older women is striking, given the richness of work by feminist sociologists, although recent research is beginning to redress this neglect.

Within the (in many ways) closely linked fields of health and social care, work which explores how older women are disadvantaged over men in respect of access to social care is exemplified by Scott's and Wenger's research around social support networks in later life. In relation to health, the authors echo Arber and Ginn and others like Graham (1984) in stating that despite a lower life expectancy, men experience better health than women do in later life. They point out that 'women live longer in poor health while older men are less likely to be limited by physical disability than women (Wenger 1987)'.

Evidence from studies which explored social support in North Wales and in Liverpool (Scott and Wenger 1995) suggest that 'older husbands rely primarily on their wives for both expressive and instrumental help, whereas older wives tend to look outside marriage for significant proportions of emotional support' (Scott and Wenger 1995, p.171).

Taking race seriously

In their book *Nursing for a Multi-ethnic Society*, Gerrish, Husband and Mackenzie (1996) make the useful point, often ignored in analyses of race and health care, that the response of post-war Britain to the 'settlement of migrant workers and to the development of minority ethnic communities has to be seen as part of the continuing process of the construction of British identity' (p.11). This is important, because in accounting for how 'race' affects health, a knowledge of the context within which health is experienced by minority ethnic communities (both collective and individual members' experiences) is essential.

The authors of this helpful text proceed to show (from a social–psychological viewpoint) how a national 'spuriously homogeneous' self-image has been constructed over the centuries, and how this image is linked with the 'invention of tradition'. They note that the assumed homogeneity actually suppresses a history rich in diversity (p.13), including the Romans, Angles, Saxons, Normans, Huguenots,

European Jews and a long history of black settlement in Britain. The authors then proceed to explain the various responses to what was seen as a potential threat to homogeneity – incoming others. Assimilation was one policy which assumed first that 'they would learn to become like us' and, second, that the 'newcomer' would be allowed to merge into the "host" society'. Assimilation failed and was, according to Gerrish, Husband and Mackenzie (1996), replaced by multiculturalism which allowed for the recognition of ethnic diversity. The problem with this policy was the focus on 'culture'. The authors write:

> Regrettably, this focus upon culture allowed the majority institutions to locate their difficulties in meeting the assumed needs of minority communities as being within the minority culture . . . minority ethnic communities were perceived to be responsible for their own failure to progress.

Again we catch a glimpse of the spectre of individualism with its emphasis on taking individual responsibility for health and other matters and its failure to address issues of power and related resource inequalities between majority and minority communities.

Ahmad (1994) gives some examples of how specific groups of people have been targeted in this way. He writes:

> In the late 1950s and 1960s medical researchers expressed fears about the incidence of tuberculosis in the recent (largely black) immigrants to Britain . . . particularly inasfar as this posed a threat for the white population. This was tempered with relief that the immigrants had shown little tendency to integrate and therefore not spread the disease to the local population. In this scenario tuberculosis became a "disease of immigrants", an imported disease, and among the many "exotic" diseases to be associated with black immigrants. (p.20)

Ahmad also mentions the 'Stop Rickets Campaign' (we refer to Pearson's comments on this campaign in Chapter 2). He reminds us that once rickets was understood to be a disease associated with poverty which was controlled by fortifying margarine with vitamin D, improvements in standards of living and universal availability of free milk to school children. He comments on how rickets then emerged as an 'Asian' disease 'explained in terms of un-British eating and living habits, and perhaps a genetic deficiency in absorbing vitamin D into the bloodstream or in synthesizing vitamin D from sunlight'. He continues:

> Vitamin D deficiency in Asian women was said to be due to the oppression of women in Asian cultures, where men insist on modest dress and impose

restrictions on women subathing. And he observes how this view of rickets fuelled the prediction that the long term answer to Asian rickets probably lies in health education and a change towards the Western diet and lifestyle. (p.21)

Gerrish, Husband and Mackenzie (1996) point out that in the late 1970s through to the mid 1980s 'multiculturalism was critiqued by members of minority ethnic communities, who deeply resented its implicit paternalism, and by political analysts, who felt it obscured the structural basis of inequality' (p.15). Antiracist strategies emerged as an alternative policy. It drew on the idea of institutionalized racism, the process by which racist ideas are appealed to in order to justify relationships, policies and practices which perpetuate inequality and the oppression of specific groups of people. However, as Gerrish, Husband and Mackenzie point out, it drew critics from both the right and left. The latter 'found it strong on rhetoric and weak on action' and the right targeted local authorities and others who embraced it as 'looney left' (p.16).

In the present political climate, antiracist strategies are manifest to a degree in equal opportunities policies. However, according to Gerrish, Husband and Mackenzie, 'while they may make explicit discrimination on racial grounds against individuals more difficult, their impact on patterns of inequality between different ethnic communities is very limited and slow' (p.17).

Connecting race and gender

Ahmad comments on how feminist critiques of patriarchy in relation to the concerns of white women such as birth control and abortion were never shared by black women (Ahmad 1994, p.25). Angela Davis (1988) makes a similar point, but conveys quite poignantly something of the complexity of the issue of abortion for black women. Commenting on the abortion rights campaign in the USA and the early 1970s when abortions were at last declared legal, she writes:

> The ranks of the abortion rights campaign did not include substantial numbers of women of color . . . .. When questions were raised . . . two explanations were commonly proposed . . . .. Women of color were overburdened by their people's fight against racism and/or they had not yet become conscious of the centrality of sexism. (p.203)

Challenging this view, she explains how black women in slavery in the USA actually practised abortion (and infanticide) not so much from a desire to be free of their pregnancies but rather because of the intolerable social conditions they indured and which they did not want their children to endure. The reasons for the seeming lack of black women's interests in the abortion campaign of the 1960s was because they did not see abortion as a stepping stone to freedom, but rather as an act of desperation.

The important point is that unilinear explanations, whether they be based on class, race, gender and age, cannot convey complexity of experience. Crenshaw writing in 1994 (pp.39–52) observes that it is difficult to analyse the multidimensionality of black women's experiences within a single-axis analysis. She is referring to the absence of patriarchy and gender in antiracist analyses and the absence of race in feminist analyses. In our discussion we have tried to convey the importance of taking difference, diversity and associated power inequalities seriously in discussing 'community'.

Taking this approach we can move away from a position where the views of minority groups are subordinated. For example, within the field of women's health there is a call for justice in the provision of health care. However, justice is experienced differently depending on whether one is a black woman or a white woman (Davis 1984, 1988; Bryan, Dadzie and Scafe 1988; Anderson 1991; Anderson *et al.* 1993). And even these categories are not homogeneous. Further factors add to the complexity of women's experiences of health, among them age, class and employment status as well as where in the world a woman lives. These and other socioeconomic factors which affect how women experience health care (Anderson 1991) are important to take into account in nursing practice, so that the experiences of a minority are not subordinated to the majority and silenced, or relegated, to the lower end of a hierarchy of knowledge about women's health needs (Williams 1996, pp.91–92) – or indeed any minority needs.

How far, then, can sociological perspectives on community help us to understand health and healthcare issues? We suggest that taking 'inequalities' into account can be helpful, in the sense that socioeconomic factors can and do affect people's access to and experiences of health. Communities are never homogeneous, and this is important to grasp when thinking about how we as nurses and other healthcare workers provide care. We have concentrated on difference in relation to socioeconomic factors such as class, age, race and gender, and we have acknowledged geographical location.

Summary

We have explored 'community', commenting on the heterogeneity of the idea. Discussion has mainly centred on inequalities in health in the community. Throughout the discussion we catch glimpses of sociological resistance to the legacy of individualism which pervades our taken-for-granted everyday thinking, and we are brought back to the point we make in the introduction to this book: the sociological critique of difference and an emphasis on 'inequalities' constitutes an important intellectual contribution to our understanding of the broader context within which we work and live, it is also importantly a political and moral standpoint. Readers may want to consider what their responses are to the implications of the critique for their practice as nurses and other healthcare workers.

References

Ahmad W.I.U. (1994) Making black people sick: 'race', ideology and health research in Ahmad W.I.U. (ed.) *'Race' and Health in Contemporary Britain*. Milton Keynes, Open University Press.

Anderson J. (1991) Immigrant women speak of chronic illness: the social construction of the devalued self. *Journal of Advanced Nursing* 16, 710–717.

Anderson J., Blue C., Holbrook A. and Ng M. (1993) On chronic illness: immigrant women in Canada's work force – a feminist perspective. *Canadian Journal of Nursing Research* 25(2), 7–22.

Anon (1994) Inaction over inequalities in health. Editorial. *British Medical Journal* 308, 1157–1178.

Arber S. (1991) 'Opening the 'black box': inequalities in women's health in Abbott P. and Payne G. (eds) *New Directions in the Sociology of Health*. Basingstoke, Falmer Press.

Arber S. and Ginn J. (1993) Gender and inequalities in health in later life. *Social Sciences for Medicine* 36(1), 33–46.

Arber S. and Ginn J. (1995) *Connecting Gender and Ageing*. Buckingham, Open University Press.

Bearon LB. (1989) No great expectations: the underpinnings of life satisfaction for older women. *Gerontologist* 29, 772–784.

Bryan B., Dadzie S. and Scafe S. (1988). *The Heart of Race: black women's lives in Britain*. London, Virago Press.

Central Statistical Office (1975) *Social Trends*, Volume 15. London, HMSO.

Cornwell J. (1986) *Hard-Earned Lives*. London, Tavistock.

Coward R. (1983) *Patriarchal Precedents*. London, Routledge and Kegan Paul.

Crenshaw K. (1994) Demarginalising the intersection of race and sex: a black feminist critique of antidiscrimination doctrine, feminist theory and anti-racist politics, in Jaggar A.M. (ed.) *Living with Contradictions*. Boulder, Colorado, Westview Press.

Davis A. (1984). *Women, Culture and Politics*. London, The Women's Press.

Davis A. (1988) *Women, Race and Class*. London, The Women's Press.

Dorling D. (1997) *Death in Britain. How local mortality rates have changed: 1950s–1990s*. Joseph Rowntree Foundation.

Finch J. and Groves D. (1983) *A Labour of Love: women, work and caring*.London, Routledge and Kegan Paul.

Freund P. and McGuire (1995) *Health, Illness and the Social Body: a critical sociology*, 2nd edn. New Jersey, Prentice Hall.

Gerrish K., Husband C. and McKenzie J. (1996) *Nursing for a Multi-ethnic Society*. Milton Keynes, Open University Press.

Goffman E. (1968) *Asylums: essays on the social situation of patients and other inmates*. Harmondsworth, Penguin (first published by Anchor, New York).

Graham H. (1984) *Women, Health and the Family.* Brighton, Sussex, Harvester Press.

Ignatief M. (1985) *The Needs of Strangers.* London, Tavistock.

Jones L. (1994) *The Social Context of Health and Health Work.* London, Macmillan.

Jootun D. and McGhee G. (1996) Why the modern community has stopped caring. *Nursing Times* 92(30), 40–41.

Nisbet R. (1967) *The Sociological Tradition.* London, Heinemann.

Phillimore P., Beattie A. and Townsend P. (1994) Widening inequality of health in Northern England, 1981–91. *British Medical Journal* 308, 1125–1129.

Richman J. (1987) *Medicine and Health.* London, Longman.

Schumacher T. (1960) *Small is Beautiful.* Harmondsworth, Penguin.

Scott A. and Wenger GC. (1995) Gender and social support systems in later life, in Arber S. and Ginn J. (eds.) *Connecting Gender with Ageing.* Milton Keynes, Open University Press, pp. 158–172.

Scull A. (1983) *Recarceration – Community Treatment and the Deviant: a radical view.* Cambridge, Polity Press.

Tonnies F. (1957) *Community and Society.* London, Harper Row.

Townsend P., Davidson N. and Whitehead M. (1990) *Inequalities in Health, the Black report, the health divide* Harmondsworth, Penguin.

Weinstein D. and Weinstein M. (1993) Simmel and the Theory of Postmodern Society in Turner B. (ed.) *Theories of Modernity and Postmodernity.* London, Sage.

Wenger, G.C. (1987) Dependence, interdependence and reciprocity after 80. *Journal of Ageing Studies* 1(4), 355–377.

Wilkinson R. (1994) Divided we fall: the poor pay the price of increased social inequality with their health. *British Medical Journal* 308, 1113–1114

Williams A. (1996) The politics of feminist ethnography. *Canadian Journal of Nursing Research* 28(1), 87–94.

Williams R. (1984) *Keywords: a dictionary of culture and society.* Harmondsworth, Penguin.

Wolft K. (1950) *The Sociology of G. Simmel.* Glencoe, IL, Free Press.

Young M. and Willmott P. (1957) *Family and Kinship in East London.* Harmondsworth, Penguin.

4

Religion

Introduction

Religions have a central concern with explanations of pain, suffering and death. It could be argued, therefore, that their importance to sociologists of health and illness is self-evident. Nevertheless, religion has been strikingly neglected by sociologists of illness. Williams (1993b), has suggested that this has been because both medicine and sociology are highly secularized and therefore regard religion as an epiphenomenon.

Where sociologists have turned their attention to religion, it has often been only to predict its demise. Meanwhile health care has become an increasingly secular domain with only vestigial remains of its religious foundations. For example, the routine of ward prayers at the start of each shift which one of the authors remembers from her nurse training is largely a thing of the past. However, as nurses in particular have come to define their interest in the patient as 'holistic', there has been a resurgence of interest in religion and spirituality. This is reflected in a proliferation of books and articles on 'spiritual' issues and guides to patients' religious beliefs and practices (e.g. McGilloway and Myco 1985; Neuberger 1994; Sampson 1982). Arguably these changes reflect both the changing role of nursing and the changing role of religion in contemporary society.

In this chapter, we will look at classical and contemporary sociological studies of religion and their application to health care. We will be concerned therefore with understanding the complex relationships between religion, society and illness in the contemporary world.

Classical sociological accounts of religion

In our discussion of the family we noted that much contemporary debate focused on the notion that the family was 'in decline' in contemporary society. We considered the rhetoric of this debate and the way in which it sought to construct a particular view of the family. Much of the sociological discussion of religion echoes these themes. The key theme which has united much sociological writing about religion is that of secularization. By secularization we mean the progressive decline of the importance of religion in the world. As we will see when we discuss death in a later chapter, many sociologists of health and illness assume that secularization is an accomplished fact but the empirical evidence to support this assertion is complex and far from clear cut.

It is important to distinguish between secularization and secularism. Whereas secularization refers to the declining significance of religion (what Max Weber described as the 'disenchantment of the world'), secularism refers to a rationalist and materialist system of thought which rejects religious beliefs as ignorant and irrational superstition. Secular rationalism draws on a philosophical distinction between 'reason' and 'faith'. Secular rationalism can be traced back to the eighteenth-century Enlightenment period, although it has earlier roots particularly in the civilization of ancient Greece.

The Enlightenment heralded a period in which science and rationality became increasingly important in society. These cultural changes accompanied the widespread social changes brought about by the Industrial Revolution. The influence of secular rationalism on classical sociological theories of religion is apparent and many of them proceed from an assumption that religion entails a suspension of reason which requires explanation. Secularist sociologists therefore seized on evidence of the decline of religion as evidence of the increasing enlightenment of the world. More recently, disillusionment with scientific rationality has led to a questioning of some of these assumptions. Such schools of thought have described themselves as 'post modernist' or 'post positivist' and are represented in nursing by theorists such as Patricia Benner.

Beckford (1989) suggests that it is impossible to disentangle the sociological view of religion from wider social theories and problems.

Classical sociologists shaped their theories about religion in response to their attempts to understand the rise of industrial capitalism and ameliorate the problems of deprivation and disharmony which they saw following in its wake. According to Beckford (1989), sociological thinking about religion has failed to keep pace with the changing nature of society and is still rooted in these classical theories. This is particularly true of the theory of secularization which has failed to appreciate that the disappearance of nineteenth-century forms of religion does not imply the disappearance of religion itself. As a starting point, therefore, we need to understand how classical nineteenth-century sociologists viewed religion and the way in which their ideas have shaped contemporary debates.

The work of Marx was typical of nineteenth-century secular rationalism in its dismissal of religious beliefs. Marx saw religion as a form of human self-alienation. Marx's ideas drew on the work of Feuerbach (1957), who described the idea of God as an alienation of the highest human powers. Humans projected their own power onto a deity and thus became estranged from their true natures. Humanity had only to see behind this disguise to grasp the illusory nature of religion. Liberation and progress would then result from the establishment of a humanist belief system. Marx concurred with Feuerbach in seeing religion as a form of alienation:

> The more the worker expends himself in work the more powerful becomes the world of objects which he creates in face of himself and the poorer he himself becomes in his inner life, the less he belongs to himself. It is just the same in religion. The more of himself man attributes to God, the less he has left of himself.
>
> (Bottomore and Rubel 1973)

For Marx, however, the source of this alienation is the economic relations of society as evidenced in the worker's relation to the fruits of his labour in the passage above. Religion is rooted in social oppression and reconciles humanity to that oppression:

> Religious suffering is at the same time an expression of real suffering and a protest against real suffering. Religion is the sigh of the oppressed creature, the sentiment of a heartless world and the soul of soulless conditions. It is the opium of the people. The abolition of religion, as the illusory happiness of men is a demand for their real happiness. The call to abandon their illusions about their condition is a call to abandon a condition which requires illusion.
>
> (Bottomore and Rubel 1973)

Marx looked forward to a society rid of oppression in which justice would be realized on earth and religion would become unnecessary.

By contrast, those writers referred to in many texts as 'consensus theorists' have stressed the functional necessity of religion. Durkheim believed that there was 'something eternal in religion', although the dynamic nature of society meant that religious forms and beliefs would change.

For Durkheim, religion was the means whereby society collectively expressed its central values and identity through ceremonials and rituals. Religion therefore promoted social cohesion and acted as a social cement. Durkheim was preoccupied with the way in which industrialization both threatened and changed the basis of social solidarity. (We have previously discussed his study of suicide in this context.) Religion would survive because:

> There can be no society which does not feel the need of upholding and reaffirming at regular intervals the collective sentiments and the collective ideas which make up its unity and its personality.
>
> (Durkheim, 1976)

Durkheim predicted that while religious institutions might decline, the functions of religion would persist. Whereas, in pre-industrial society, religious worship was largely collective in modern society, religion would become individualized. Religion would express the sacredness inherent in each individual as an expression of the moral community. Durkheim's ideas have found expression in the work of contemporary sociologists who have argued that religious beliefs have become increasingly personal and privatized (Luckmann, 1967).

Thus, many functionalist authors would argue that religion has not declined, but persists in new forms. This is countered by proponents of the secularization thesis who argue that functionalist definitions of religion are so all embracing that they include ideas and beliefs that ordinary people would not recognize as religious (Bruce, 1996).

Proponents of the secularization thesis undoubtedly draw many of their ideas from the work of Max Weber, in particular his concern with the process of rationalization.

Weber was concerned both with the way in which society shaped religious ideas and also with the way in which religious ideas influenced society. These concerns are expressed in particular in his best known study on the relationship between Protestantism and the rise of capitalism (Weber, 1974). In Weber's discussion of the social psychology of religion, Weber says much that is of interest to sociologists of illness about the way in which religions construct explanations of suffering and death. Such justifications and mitigations of suffering are described as theodicies.

The idea of suffering as a form of punishment is of profound importance in almost all religious traditions. Weber says that the fortunate are not content with good fortune alone, but need to believe that they have a right to be fortunate. Thus, wealth, power and good health are legitimated by the 'theory of good fortune', and suffering is treated as a sign of 'odiousness in the eyes of the Gods'. (These ideas find particular expression in the Judaeo-Christian tradition in the Book of Job.)

Thus, the possessor of good fortune consoles her/his conscience with the belief that she/he deserves it as much as the unfortunate deserve their misery. The persistence however of injustice and undeserved suffering lead to the idea of a saviour or redeemer who will right all wrongs by either 'the return of good fortune in this world or the security of happiness in the next world' (Gerth and Wright Mills 1970).

Thus, new theodicies emerge which promise salvation to the suffering. Examples include the Christian Messiah and the Cult of Krishna in Hinduism.

Weber saw the modern world as characterized by increasing rationalization. The spread of rationality pushed the need for explanations of suffering to the margins of our consciousness. Rationality had 'demystified' the world. In some senses nineteenth-century sociologists could be seen as offering secular versions of salvation through their preoccupation with righting social evils and creating conditions of social justice.

Science, however, can explain how events such as sickness occur, but it is limited in its explanations of why such events occur. According to Clark:

> How and why questions seem therefore to keep alive the distinction between science and religion. When related to some conditions of human misfortune – say

sickness – they may be posed as the opposition between two problems "how is my condition caused" and "why is this happening to me". Where does the individual find answers to these "why" questions?

(Clark, 1982)

How individuals find meaning in suffering is a key to understanding the individual's response to illness. Weber's ideas suggest that these 'why' questions are marginalized. The rise of modern medicine is one instance of the increasing rationalization of the world, with its central focus on how illness is caused and its location of the source of illness in the physiology of the individual.

However, for Weber in contrast to some of his more recent followers:

The disenchantment of the world, the calculability of everything was more of a tendency than an accomplished fact.

(Beckford, 1989)

there would always be counter tendencies and areas of social life which resisted the process of rationalization. Weber utilized the concept of charisma to explain the rise of new religious and social movements not based on rational or traditional authority.

Charismatic authority is wielded by an individual who is able to achieve power through revelation, magical power or simply force of personality. Charismatic authority implies the breakdown of existing systems of authority whether rational or traditional and therefore entails the creation of new and revolutionary social, political or religious movements. By its very nature, charismatic authority is short lived and charisma becomes 'routinized' as the movement settles down and becomes institutionalized. James and Field (1992) have analysed the 'routinisation of charisma' in the growing bureaucratization of the hospice movement.

Weber's concept of charisma implied that religions would not decline inexorably. New religions would arise with charismatic leaders and existing religions would experience periods of charismatic revival.

The significance of the concept of charisma has been variously interpreted. For some, charismatic religions are mere punctuation points in the irreversible 'disenchantment of the world', whereas, for others, they show the potential of religious movements to overthrow the existing social order. We can follow some of these classical sociological ideas into studies of contemporary religion.

Religion: declining or changing?

Sociologists have looked for evidence of the declining or changing fortunes of religion in three ways:

1. Patterns of religious membership and affiliation.
2. Patterns of religious belief.
3. The influence of religion on major social institutions.

Changing forms of religious affiliation

Changing patterns of religious affiliation have to be considered in relation to the different types of religious organizations which exist in contemporary UK society. Sociologists have developed a number of typologies of religious organizations. Churches are large scale, formal organizations with professional clergy, which are often highly bureaucratic. They may be closely allied to the state as in the case of the Church of England or the Catholic church in Eire. The Church of England has suffered a dramatic decline in attendance with only 1.8 million attending regularly in 1992 (Davie 1994a), yet it is still the church to which the majority (25.5 million of the population) claim allegiance. Most only attend church for significant events such as baptisms, weddings, funerals and Christmas. Some historians believe that this loose affiliation with the church reflects traditional patterns of 'folk' religion which were only temporarily interrupted by a period of evangelism in the Victorian era. Bruce (1996), on the other hand, has argued that a corresponding decline in infant baptism supports the existence of a process of inexorable secularization. Ironically, this decline is at least in part due to the increasing evangelism of the remaining active church membership. Many churches have become more exclusive, imposing tests of faith and loyalty on those who seek baptism of their infants or marriage in church that would have been unheard of 50 years ago.

In spite of a general decline in active church membership, there remain significant local and regional differences. Congregations still thrive in some areas, particularly rural areas and provinces such as Northern Ireland. Furthermore, immigrant communities show no signs of adopting the rather lukewarm attitude to religion characteristic of their host country. Bruce (1996) argues that religion has an important role in expressing ethnic and cultural identity and that in many of these situations, it is used as a 'cultural defence'.

The rather dramatic evidence of a decline in active church membership has fuelled arguments in favour of the secularization thesis. The evidence is visible to all as throughout our towns and cities as redundant churches and chapels are converted into shops, warehouses and bingo halls. The rather more buoyant fortunes of other religious groups have sometimes gone unnoticed, yet few towns of a significant size have not seen the erection of a Kingdom Hall by their local Jehovah's Witnesses.

Sectarian groups such as the Jehovah's Witnesses have usually arisen in radical protest against existing religions often through a charismatic leader. They are highly organized groups which see themselves as true believers and draw strong boundaries between 'them' and 'us'. Many believe that the end of the world is nigh and only they will be saved. Some modern sects have been remarkably successful in exploiting mass communications and marketing techniques to spread their message (Schmalz 1994). Some of the larger sects such as the Mormons and Jehovah's Witnesses owe much of their success to their use of the techniques of successful business corporations, which is an irony given their ostensible rejection of secular rationalism.

Niebuhr (1929) argued that after a period of time, sects would 'cool down' and become more established and tolerant of other religions. He described these groups as denominations. Denominational groups such as the Methodists have suffered very serious declines in membership. It may be that newer sects are learning this lesson and instituting mechanisms for maintaining a sectarian identity and boundaries between members and outsiders. A good example of this strategy of boundary maintenance is the decision of the Jehovah's Witnesses to institute a taboo on blood transfusions in the post-war period (Singelenberg, 1990).

The rising fortunes of sectarian groups can be related in part to their successful methods of discipline and boundary maintenance in maintaining their membership. They can also be understood in relation to the rise of evangelism and religious fundamentalism which stands in contrast and reaction to increasing secularism.

Fundamentalism was a term originally applied to the defence of Protestant orthodoxy against modern scientific thought, particularly the theory of evolution. The term has come to be applied more generally to religious movements which defend religious orthodoxy against the encroachments of contemporary culture (Marty and Scott Appleby 1993). Fundamentalist movements have arisen in all parts of the world and in all religious traditions. Key features of fundamentalist movements include:

> A general hostility towards a rationalist post-Enlightenment view of the world; an emphasis on supernatural intervention in daily mundane affairs; a restored patriarchy under a charismatic leader who draws his legitimacy from God . . . initial intransigence, born of millennial expectations followed (when the millennium fails to materialise) by some form of accommodation or bargaining with the larger world; a tendency to "fight back" against the current of the times while appropriating those aspects of contemporary culture that seem necessary or desirable.
>
> (Ruthuen 1993)

The globalization of social life brings us into increasing contact with other religious traditions. The fundamentalist response to making sense of increasingly fragmented world views is to choose one all-encompassing view of the world and stick with it. Fundamentalists also see themselves as fighting back against the encroachments of secular rationalism and may become increasingly interested in obtaining secular power to achieve their ends. Robertson (1989) sees globalization as leading to the politicization of religion and the religionization of politics. Davie (1994b) predicts a growth of intransigent and competing fundamentalisms. We can predict from this a growth in conflicts between religious groups and civic society such as the Waco siege and the Sarin gas attacks by the Aum cult in Japan.

While for some the response to changing times has been found in the fierce allegiance of sectarianism, there has been another quite different response. One response to the variety of religious ideas and beliefs on offer in a global society is to select your own personal package. Davie (1994a) has described this phenomenon as 'supermarket religion'. Many authors have described the rise of a loose network of religious or quasi-religious organizations and practices which have been described as the 'new age movement' or 'cultic milieu'.

Although these new religious movements or 'cults' have attracted negative media attention in recent years due to their supposed ability to 'brainwash' their members, research suggests that membership is short lived and individuals attracted to these movements can be described as 'seekers' who pursue a variety of unorthodox religious beliefs and practices often simultaneously (Barker 1989).

Heelas (1993a and 1996) has borrowed the term of the 'new age' to refer to the cultic milieu, he and others have noted some key features of this religious milieu. The first is its eclecticism, religious groups draw on a wide variety of religious ideas and symbols without worrying very much about their logical connections or contradictions. Lyon (1993) has with good reason described the new age movement as 'a bit of a circus'. Loose connections are made through the use of metaphors or umbrella terms such as 'energy', 'balance' and 'holism' (Bruce 1996).

For Heelas (1993b), the central theme of the new age is the 'sacralisation of the self'. This echoes Durkheim's earlier view that religion would come to symbolize the sacredness of the individual. The new age has been linked to a culture of 'expressivism' (Walter 1993) in which the goal of self-realization becomes paramount. This culture (also described by Lasch (1979) as 'narcissism') finds its secular expression in humanistic psychology and many contemporary forms of psychotherapy and counselling. In the 'self-religions' these ideas are extended, we should not only seek to 'find ourselves', but to find God within ourselves. Social relations are seen as oppressive of 'authenticity' or 'true spirit'. Bruce (1996) sees the new age as the apotheosis of a consumerist and individualistic society. He argues that it is a 'grand irony' that such groups regard themselves as 'alternative', because they are the perfect product of their time. The new age is the 'acme of consumerism', it is 'individualism raised to a new plane'. It leads individuals to suppose that 'by knowing oneself, we can know everything'.

New age movements take different forms and encompass religious groups and communities as well as individual therapists and practitioners. Many of the beliefs and practices of the 'new age' have entered mainstream culture and this is particularly true of 'alternative' therapies such as aromatherapy which have spawned an enormous range of consumer products. We will return to the link between the 'new age', complementary therapies and nursing later.

Believing without belonging

We have painted a picture of declining church membership coupled with some growth areas, in particular, sectarian and fundamentalist movements and new age movements. Empirical studies have consistently reported high levels of religious belief in spite of declining church membership. A survey in 1990 found that 71% of the UK population believed in God, 25% were undecided and only 4% claimed to be atheists (Davie 1994b).

Three themes can be identified in sociological explanations of 'believing without belonging'. First, the theme of 'self-religions' identified with earlier Durkheimian ideas and described in Luckmann's (1967) work as 'privatised' systems of religion. Perhaps the 'new age' can be seen as the creation of a consumer culture for these privatized religious systems.

Linked to this sociologists have identified a general decline in membership of communal organizations. Declining church membership can be seen as a reflection of declining communal values rather than declining religious values and no different from the decline of football clubs, trade unions, etc. (Davie 1994a).

Finally, some social historians have talked of 'common' or 'folk' religion instead of 'private' religion. The existence of high levels of belief alongside low levels of practice are seen as characteristic of religion before the Industrial Revolution (Davie 1994a). Folk traditions and informal practices existing outside formal structures are fairly persistent (Clark 1982; Davie 1994a). These 'unofficial' religious practices draw on shared meanings and are not entirely personal. Such beliefs may not be prominent in everyday life, but may be drawn on at times of transition or crisis, such as childbirth, illness and death. Other authors have described this as the 'God of the gaps', to be consulted when other strategies have failed (Abercrombie *et al.* 1970).

Declining religious influence

If most areas of our life are controlled by secular institutions and our God is a 'God of the gaps', then religion has little influence in our lives whatever the faith we profess. One area in which this argument has been stated particularly forcibly has been in the literature on the growing influence of medical authority or 'medicalisation'.

Freidson (1970) claimed that:

> the hospital is succeeding the church and the parliament as the archetypical institution of Western culture

and Zola (1972) suggested that:

> medicine expands its jurisdiction to cover more and more areas once reserved for law and religion.

We can hear resonances of Weber's work on the 'iron cage' of rationality here. Turner (1987) sees the growth of western rationality as having three dimensions. First, the process of secularization, second the growing importance of science and technology, and finally (echoing the work of Foucault), the increasing importance of 'systems of individual discipline and regulation by bureaucratic agencies related to the nation state'. Medicine provides us with an example of these processes:

> Put simply, the doctor has replaced the priest as the custodian of social values. The panoply of ecclesiastical institutions of regulation have been transferred through the evolution of scientific medicine to a panoptic collection of localised agencies of surveillance and control.
>
> (Turner 1987)

In summing up, we can say that sociological studies of contemporary religion have produced a complex picture of competing trends. While there is evidence of declining church membership and the declining institutional influence of religion, there is also evidence of a high level of religious belief independent of church organizations. For some this represents the pursuit of 'self realization', through engaging in therapies and rituals variously described as 'new age' or 'cultic'. For others, religion is a more marginal part of existence more properly described as a 'God of the gaps'. At the same time, there is a definite reaction to secularization with an increase in sectarian groups offering a fundamentalist outlook on life.

Clearly, this complex pattern of contemporary religious life has an impact on the response of individuals to illness, suffering and death, which is worthy of our attention. In addition, we may wish to consider the effect of these cultural influences on nursing.

Religion, illness and health

One factor which has interested a number of sociologists is the apparent relationship between religious affiliation and health. Put simply, the religious tend to live longer and be more healthy (Jarvis and Northcutt 1987; Levin 1994). Explanations have focused on the way in which religions offer social support and promote a healthy lifestyle following a conventional functionalist perspective. Interestingly, a recent study of Kibbutzim found that members of religious Kibbutzim were healthier than members of secular kibbutzim, suggesting that the content of beliefs may also be important (Anson *et al.* 1991). This brings us back to the question of theodicy and the role of religion in beliefs about health, illness and suffering.

In spite of the detailed attention which has been paid to lay concepts of health in recent years, very little attention has been paid within this literature to religious beliefs. Williams (1993b) has suggested that the moral and religious components of health beliefs are easily overlooked by the researcher.

Radley and Billig (1996) suggest that public accounts of illness reflect the speaker's concern with the medical authorities against whose criteria their statements will be judged. If religion has indeed become privatized we would expect religious concerns to be less prominent in accounts which are addressed to what is seen as a secular authority.

Williams (1990) described a 'Protestant legacy' in the accounts of health given by his Scottish respondents. Popular moral conceptions of health reflected Protestant theological debates. His respondents expressed views of health and illness which were close to Weber's 'theodicy of good fortune'.

The healthy owed their good fortune to a hardworking and virtuous existence, whereas the sick had 'brought in on themselves'. Blaxter (1993) noted similar moral views of illness and a sense of guilt among respondents who 'gave in' to sickness. In Blaxter's respondents, good health was so clearly synonymous with virtue that respondents claimed to be healthy even when this flew in the face of all the available evidence. One respondent recounting the early death of most of her close relatives concluded 'We were a healthy family'.

Williams (1993a) has described the career of the chronically sick in terms of the pursuit of virtue as they strive to assert themselves as morally blameless in spite of the stigma of their condition. Crawford (1980) suggests that current concerns with 'positive health' and 'healthy lifestyles' have extended this moral discourse into the lives of the healthy and we can see this as a continuation of the Protestant legacy in secular form.

The Judaeo-Christian tradition contains a legacy of religious ideas which place responsibility for health on the individual and see good health as a reward for a virtuous life. These ideas lead to a deep-rooted resistance to accepting the social causes of ill-health (Blaxter 1990). Similar beliefs may exist in other religious traditions and affect the individuals' response to illness (Agraval and Dalal 1993). There is clearly much more to be learned about the effect of various religious traditions on belief about health and illness and future research in this area is needed.

As regards recent changes in religions in our own society summarized earlier, we can draw out a number of implications for health care.

First, there are increasing numbers of people who are only nominally religious and whose beliefs are informal and privatized. Such individuals may only turn to religion in times of personal crisis, but their beliefs about health and illness may be influenced by religious traditions with which they have only a tenuous connection. In studies by Williams and others of health beliefs, a Protestant version of the 'theodicy of good fortune' seems to be a common set of beliefs. Second, the growth of fundamentalist groups which are often sectarian in organization presents new challenges for healthcare workers. Fundamentalism is, by its nature, in opposition to secular rationalism. Medicine is an area of secular rationalism most likely to conflict with fundamentalist groups through its involvement in issues of life, death and sexual morality.

Fundamentalist groups have become increasingly involved in debates about contraception, abortion and genetic medicine and conflicts in these areas seem bound to increase. Additionally, some sectarian groups prohibit specific medical practices, such as the Jehovah's Witnesses ban on blood transfusions. The sociological and psychological literature on sectarian groups and new religious movements is polarized between psychologists and psychiatrists who claim that these groups exercise techniques of brainwashing and 'mind control' (West 1993) and a more liberal view that individuals generally enter and leave these groups of their own free will (Barker 1989). An intermediate position is taken by some authors suggesting that the social pressures of sect membership affect the validity of an individual's judgement. This applies particularly to informed consent and refusal of treatment (Wright 1991; Young and Griffith 1992).

If, as Davie (1994b) suggests, we may become a world of 'competing fundamentalisms', current medical ethical guidelines based on assumptions of religious toleration and individual freedom may be put under increasing strain and may be unable to deal with the pressures of such a changing social context.

Religion, the 'New Age' and nursing

We have also discussed the growth of 'new age' or 'designer' religion. Nursing has traditionally had strong associations with religion. The recent popularity of new age ideas in nursing, which we will explore in this section, may well reflect a contemporary version of this traditional link between nursing and religion.

As noted earlier, the ideas of new age religions are closely linked to ideas of self-realization associated with humanistic psychologists such as Abraham Maslow. New age ideas are therefore linked to a particular discourse about health and illness which has found recent expression in nursing through its interest in 'holism' and the subjective world of the patient. (We will explore this discourse in more detail in a later chapter.)

This interest in new age ideas in nursing takes a number of forms. First, some nursing theorists, such as Rosemary Parse and Martha Rogers, make explicit use of new age ideas in their work, exploring concepts such as 'transcendence', 'four-dimensionality' and 'energy fields'. Second, nurses have become increasingly interested in the spiritual aspects of nursing care and ideas about spirituality are often linked to existential psychology (Harrison and Burnard 1993; Barber 1996). Finally, there is an enormous popular interest in complementary therapies in nursing. Many of these derive their philosophical bases from new age religions and have been described by Bruce (1996) as 'client cults'.

It is worth considering for a moment the particular discourse about health which is implicit in these developments. New age beliefs place responsibility for health on the individual often in a quite radical way. One best-selling alternative health manual claims that all 'so called illnesses' are self-inflicted and are due to negative thoughts and emotions (Hay 1988). In many self-religions quasi-magical powers are claimed for adherents to these ideas and individuals are expected to cure themselves through faith and an effort of will. In some cases, these quasi-magical beliefs have penetrated nursing theory and practice where they sit uncomfortably alongside scientific orthodoxy.

It is worth noting that these beliefs again reflect the 'theodicy of good fortune'. The individual is again responsible for her/his happiness or woe. Such discourses reflect a direct repudiation of the social causes of ill health. Indeed the holistic model employed here is not the 'bio-psychosocial' model, but the 'mind, body, spirit'. Such authors are relentlessly individualistic, they seek communion with the cosmos, but not with their local community.

Some nursing writers have lamented the way in which nursing has moved from an earlier religious tradition of 'service' and 'vocation' towards the 'self-religions' (Bradshaw 1994). We can also link this change to a move towards words rather than deeds as nursing tries to make concepts of 'holism' and the 'nurse–patient relationship' central to its endeavours. It is perhaps an irony that nurses are turning to complementary therapies such as therapeutic touch and aroma-therapy, to put them in touch with the patient at a time when they are turning their backs on physical care and increasingly allowing it to be carried out by unqualified staff.

References

Abercrombie N., Baker J., Brett S. and Foster J. (1970) Superstition and Religion: the God of the gaps, in Martin D. and Hill M. (eds) *A Sociological Yearbook of Religion*. London, SCM.

Anson O., Levenson A., Maoz B. and Bonneh D.Y. (1991) Religious community, individual religiosity and health: a tale of two kibbutzim. *Sociology* 25(1), 119–113.

Agrawal M. and Dalal A (1993). Beliefs about the world and recovery from myocardial infarction. *Journal of Social Psychology* 133(3), 385–394.

Barber P. (1996) Social symbolism of health: the notion of the soul in professional care, in Perry A. (ed.) *Insights from Sociology*. London, Arnold.

Barker E. (1989) *New Religious Movements: a practical introduction*. London, HMSO.

Beckford J. (1989) *Religion and Advanced Industrial Society*. London, Unwin Hyman.

Blaxter M. (1990) *Health and Lifestyles*. London, Routledge.

Blaxter M. (1993) 'Why do the victims blame themselves?', in Radley A. (ed.) *Worlds of Illness: biographical and cultural perspectives on health and disease*. London, Routledge.

Bottomore T.B. and Rubel M. (1973) Karl Marx, in *Selected Writings in Sociology and Social Philosophy*. Penguin Books, Harmondsworth.

Bradshaw A. (1994) *Lighting the Lamp: the spiritual dimension of nursing care*. London, Scutari.

Bruce S. (1996) *Religion in the Modern World: from Cathedrals to cults*. Oxford, Oxford University Press.

Clark D. (1982) *Between Pulpit and Pew: folk religion in a North Yorkshire fishing village*. Cambridge, Cambridge University Press.

Crawford R. (1980) Healthism and the medicalisation of everyday life. *International Journal of Health Services* 10(3), 365–80

Davie G. (1994a) *Religion in Britain since 1945: believing without belonging*. Oxford, Blackwell.

Davie G. (1994b) Religion in post-war Britain: a sociological view, in Obelkevich J. and Catterall P. (eds) *'Understanding Post-War British Society*. London, Routledge.

Durkheim E. (1976) *The Elementary Forms of Religious Life.* 1859–1917. London, Allen and Unwin.

Feuerbach L. (1957) *Essences of Christianity.* New York, Harper.

Freidson E. (1970) Profession of Medicine. New York, Dodd, Mead and Co.

Gerth H.H. and Wright Mills C. (eds) (1970) *From Max Weber: essays in sociology.* London, Routledge.

Hay L. (1988) *You Can Heal Your Life.* London, Eden Grove Editions.

Harrison J. and Burnard P. (1993) *Spirituality and Nursing Practice.* Avebury, Aldershot.

Heelas P. (1993a) The new age in cultural context: the pre-modern, the modern and the post-modern. *Religion* 23 103–111.

Heelas P. (1993b) The sacralisation of the self and new age capitalism, in Abercrombie N. and Ward A. (eds) *Social Change in Contemporary Society.* Cambridge, Polity.

Heelas P. (1996) *The New Age Movement, Celebrating the Self and the Sacralisation of Modernity.* Cambridge, MA, Blackwell.

James N. and Field D. (1992) The routinisation of hospice: charisma and bureaucratisation. *Social Science and Medicine* 34, 1363–1375.

Jarvis G.K. and Northcott H.D. (1987) Religion and differences in morbidity and mortality. *Social Science and Medicine* 25(7), 813–824.

Lasch C. (1979) *The Culture of Narcissism.* London, Abacus.

Levin J. (1994) Religion and health: is there an association? *Social Science and Medicine* 38(11), 1475–1482.

Luckmann T. (1967) *The invisible religion.* New York, Macmillan.

Lyon D. (1993) A bit of a circus: notes on postmodernity and new age. *Religion,* 23, 117–126.

Marty M.E. and Scott Appleby R. (1993) *Fundamentalism Observed.* Chicago, Chicago University Press.

McGilloway D. and Myco F. (1985) *Nuring and Spiritual Care*. London, Harper and Row.

Neuberger J. (1994) *Caring for Dying People of Different Faiths*. London, Mosby.

Niebuhr H.R. (1929) *The Social Sources of Denominationalism*. New York, Henry Holt.

Radley A. and Billig M. (1996) Accounts of health and illness: dilemmas and representations. *Sociology of Health and Illness* 18(2), 220–240.

Robertson R. (1989) Globalisation, politics and religion, in Beckford J. and Luckmann T. (eds) *The Changing Face of Religion*. London, Sage.

Ruthuen M. (1993) The audio-vision of God. *The Guardian* Saturday May 1st.

Sampson C. (1982) *The Neglected Ethic: cultural and religious factors in the care of patients*. London, McGraw Hill.

Schmalz M.N. (1994) When Festinger fails: prophecy and the watch tower. *Religion* 24, 293–308.

Singelenberg R. (1990) The blood transfusion taboo of Jehovah's Witnesses: origin, development and function of a controversial doctrine. *Social Science and Medicine* 31(4), 515–523.

Turner B.S. (1987) *Medical Power and Social Knowledge*. London, Sage.

Walter T. (1993) Death in the new age. *Religion* 23, 127–145.

Weber M. (1974) 12th Impression, *The Protestant Ethic and the Spirit of Capitalism*. London, Unwin University Books.

West L.J. (1993) A psychiatric overview of cult related phenomena. *Journal of the American Academy of Psychoanalysis* 21(1), 1–19.

Williams G. (1993) Chronic Illness and the pursuit of virtue in everyday life, in Radley A. (ed) *Worlds of Illness Biographical and Cultural Perspectives on Health and Disease*. London, Routledge.

Williams R. (1990) *A Protestant Legacy: attitudes to death and illness among older Aberdonians.* Oxford, Oxford University Press.

Williams R. (1993) Religion and Illness, in Radley A. (ed) *Worlds of Illness Biographical and Cultural Perspectives on Health and Disease.* London, Routledge.

Wright S.A. (1991) Reconceptualising cult coercion and withdrawal: a comparative analysis of divorce and apostasy. *Social Forces* 70(1), 125–145.

Young J.L. and Griffith E.H. (1992) A critical evaluation of coercive persuasion as used in the assessment of cults. *Behavioural Sciences and the Law* 10, 89–101.

Zola I.K. (1972) Medicine as an institution of social control. *Sociological Review* 20(4), 487–504.

Part Two

Sociological Perspectives on Nursing and Health

5

Nursing and Working

In this chapter we explore nursing as a form of work and examine changes in nursing work in the context of changes in work and work organization in society.

What is work?

According to Giddens:

> Work may be defined as the carrying out of tasks involving the expenditure of mental and physical effort which has as its objective the production of goods and services that cater to human needs. (1997, p.307)

This all-encompassing definition does not distinguish between paid work (employment) and unpaid work that takes place outside the formal context of the labour market. A central feature of contemporary society is its complex division of labour. Whereas in pre-industrial societies households often produced most of their own goods and services, in contemporary British society, vast areas of work are organized into specialized jobs for which individuals receive wages. The structured inequalities in society which we have noted in a previous chapter largely centre around a person's status in paid work.

Boundaries of work and employment

The centrality of the industrial division of labour in society should not blind us to the fact that many goods and services are still produced outside formal employment. It is estimated, for example, that if unpaid domestic work was paid for at the same average rate as paid employment, then the value of this work to Britain can be calculated as 122% of gross domestic production (*The Guardian* 1997). Most of this unpaid work takes place in families, households and neighbourhoods, and the majority of it is carried out by women (Oakley 1976, Graham 1984).

Our role as nurses alerts us to the fragile boundary between paid employment and unpaid work, particularly where women's work is concerned. Nurses produce a human service, but the fact that most of the tasks which we carry out in our daily employment are being carried out somewhere by an unpaid carer causes difficulties when we wish to claim special expertise and professional status. The increased throughput of hospital patients and renewed emphasis on 'community care' has intensified the pressures to move patients from paid to unpaid care. This has been driven by the continuing pressure to reduce health spending. Boundaries between unpaid work and paid employment are constantly shifting and we will go on to explore the impact of these boundary changes on the occupational identity of nursing later in our discussion.

Work and organizations

Most contemporary work takes place within organizations and a number of different themes emerge from the sociological study of organizations which are relevant to a discussion of contemporary nursing work.

The most important classical sociological study of organizations was Max Weber's work on bureaucracy (Gerth and Wright Mills 1970). The word bureaucracy comes from a French word referring to a kind of baize cloth used to cover desks and means, literally, the rule of those who sit behind desks. The term bureaucracy has always had negative connotations and Giddens (1997) quotes the French novelist Honore' de Balzac who described bureaucracy as 'the giant power wielded by pygmies'.

Weber thought the rise of bureaucracy was inevitable. He saw it as the form of rational administration most suited to large-scale social systems. Weber identified the following characteristics as typical of bureaucratic systems:

1. There are fixed rules governing all areas of activity. Rules are more or less exhaustive and can be learned.
2. There is a clear-cut hierarchy with clear lines of accountability.
3. The management of the modern organization is based upon written documents.
4. Officials are full time and salaried and their work is governed by formal training and examinations.
5. There is a clear separation between the individual's private life and working life.

Weber believed that bureaucratic organizations had advantages in terms of efficiency because they were governed by strict and impartial rules and procedures. This prevented individuals from using the organization to promote their own personal interests by, for example, promoting their kinfolk into positions of power regardless of their ability. In theory, at least in bureaucracies, open competition and formal rules of employment mean the appointment of the best person for the job.

Weber recognized that bureaucracies could have unintended negative consequences such as inflexibility and dehumanization and he talked pessimistically about the 'iron cage' of rationality in his work. To appreciate the negative consequences of bureaucratic systems we have only to turn to sociological studies of institutional life such as Goffman's work on asylums (1968).

Weber did, however, apparently believe that the formal rules and procedures which he identified in bureaucratic organizations would actually govern the activities of that organization. Thus the stated objectives of an organization should, in reality, drive the working practices of people within the organization.

In contrast to Weber's view, many studies have identified the importance of informal working practices. Wadel (1979) describes the hidden work within work organizations. It is informal activities which maintain good working relationships and keep the organization running smoothly. This hidden work is often seen as non-work by managers, and yet without it no organization would function. The very existence of 'working to rule' as a form of industrial action testifies to the importance of informal work. Few hospitals would survive very long if nurses only did what was described in their job descriptions.

Herzferd (1992) suggests that a major goal of those working in bureaucracies is their own survival within the organization. The formal language of bureaucracies should not blind us to the fact that powerful interest groups still operate within organizations to protect their own interests and individuals in positions of power can still use that power to pursue their own ends. This may explain why inequalities of class, gender and race persist in organizations with explicit equal opportunities policies. Formal rules and procedures can be a mask to disguise the pursuit of self-interest or sectional advantage. Thompson and Machugh (1990) argue that the fact that managers have appropriated the language of rationality (using terms such as 'rationalization' instead of 'cuts') does not mean that their decisions are either rational or disinterested.

Herzfeld uses the term 'secular theodicies' to describe the explanations which people construct to explain their failures and humiliations in the hands of bureaucratic organizations. The stereotype of the faceless bureaucrat is one to which both the official and the citizen can appeal. The citizen justifies his defeat by fatalistically remarking that you 'can't beat the system'. Bureaucrats absolve themselves from personal responsibility by also blaming 'the system'. This convention allows officials to wield power while evading responsibility. For example, Nazism erected a massive bureaucratic system of genocide in which everyone could claim to be 'only doing their job'. Herzfeld inverts Weber's chain of bureaucratic accountability, power is the right to be unaccountable. The chief executive of an organization described by his employees as 'Mr Teflon' because nothing sticks to him is the embodiment of this principle.

Weber's ideal type of bureaucracy identified some important properties of formal organizations, but failed to take account of what actually happens behind the scenes in real organizations. In an attempt to get to grips with the more intangible aspects of organizational life, some researchers have turned to the study of organizational culture. Borrowing from the work of Durkheim, they see organizational culture as the 'collective consciousness' of the organization. Many recent management theorists have suggested that effective leadership in an organization involves manipulating and directing organizational culture. The idea that it is possible to create a unified 'corporate culture' is naive and ignores the major conflicts of values that exist within most organizations. These are at their most acute in organizations employing professionals such as doctors and nurses who have their own explicit value systems (Mackay 1993). It may be more helpful to see an organization as a form of negotiated order in which groups and individuals contest for position with varying amounts of power and patronage at their disposal. The balance of power between different interest groups is often precarious and shifting. It is influenced by wider social, economic and political forces. For example, recent changes in health care have weakened the power of doctors *vis-à-vis* health service managers. In the following discussion on the control of work, this shifting organizational context is an important background to our discussion.

The industrial division of labour: Taylorism and Fordism

We have noted that a key feature of contemporary society is the industrial division of labour. Individuals work in highly specialized employment, often in large-scale organizations such as the NHS. The popular picture of the Industrial Revolution is of a time of technological change when great inventions such as the steam engine and the Spinning Jenny revolutionized the production of goods and services. More revolutionary was the change in the social organization of work effected by the introduction of the factory system (Thompson 1968). Prior to the creation of mills and factories the worker followed the production process from start to finish. The weaver, for example, produced a piece of cloth for sale in the local Piece Hall. Following industrialization the production process was divided into a series of tasks completed by different workers under the control of the factory manager.

Early exponents of the industrial division of labour such as Adam Smith noted the increase in production that this new style of organizing work could achieve. In the 1830s Charles Babbage also proposed that the factory system reduced the skill required of individual workers and thus weakened their bargaining powers, reducing the costs of labour. He proposed the 'Babbage principle', under which progress is measured by the extent to which the tasks of workers can be 'simplified and integrated' with the tasks of other workers (Giddens 1997).

The aim therefore of the factory manager was to exert discipline over the worker to ensure that maximum profit was extracted from their labours. Conflict and bargaining between worker and employer came to centre around the concept of a fair day's work for a fair day's pay. Initially industrial discipline was Draconian and was resisted by the populace with early mills employing mainly women and children. According to Hammond and Hammond (1949):

> In the modern world most people have to adapt themselves to some kind of discipline, and to observe other people's time-tables, to do other people's sums, or to work under other people's orders, but we have to remember that the population that was flung into the brutal rhythm of the factory had earned its living in relative freedom, and that the discipline of the early factory was particularly savage . . .. No economist of the day, in estimating the gains and the losses of factory employment ever allowed for the strain and violence a man suffered in his feelings when he passed from a life in which he could smoke or eat, or dig or sleep as he pleased to one in which somebody turned the key on him and for fourteen hours a day he had not even the right to whistle. (1949, p.33)

The emphasis on the control and strict management of tasks in the new industrial system had its influence on the creation of modern nursing at the end of the nineteenth century. The activity of nursing had been carried out historically as now by a mixture of paid work and neighbourhood or family care. Paid nursing was largely carried out by members of the servant class described by Dingwall, Rafferty and Webster (1988) as 'handywomen'. Late nineteenth-century nursing reformers such as Florence Nightingale and Mrs Bedford Fenwick described such care as at best inept and at worst immoral. Nursing reformers wished to bring a new organization and discipline to nursing based on principles of hygiene and efficiency. These reforms were also born out of a concern about the social effects of industrialization. Fears of crime, revolution and disease led to a pressing concern with the moral welfare of the industrial classes. Nursing reformers saw opportunities for upper-class spinsters to remoralize the labouring classes through their leadership of nursing. Used to disciplining domestic servants these women could impose a new moral and social order on nursing. Laws of hygiene would combine with laws of conduct, cleanliness was next to Godliness.

This was a period in which techniques of social control proliferated and the discipline of the factory was extended to the treatment of the socially deviant or incompetent. Prisons, workhouses, asylums and other specialized institutions for the indigent were created. The inmates of such institutions were expected to learn new habits of order and discipline and nurses were to play a major role in the creation of this new moral order. Surveillance also extended into the community with the creation of health visitors to bring the new laws of hygiene to the poor in their homes.

The ideas that informed the creation of contemporary nursing were a curious hybrid of moral puritanism and industrial efficiency. Industrial systems of management have been described as 'low trust' systems. Tasks are rigidly prescribed and closely supervised and the worker has little autonomy of action. A low trust system in nursing combined the practical with the moral surveillance of the nurse. The rigid demarcation and monitoring of duties, which came to be known as the 'task allocation' system, was an aspect of this. The concept of a fair day's work for a fair day's pay became central to nursing and was largely measured in terms of physical labour. The good nurse 'pulls her weight' (Clarke 1978).

Taylorism

The most developed expression of the industrial division of labour can be found in the work of Frederick Winslow Taylor. Taylor's system of 'scientific management' involved breaking tasks down to their smallest components, these could then be measured to establish the quickest and most efficient means to complete that task which Taylor described as the 'one best way' (Taylor 1947). Taylorist systems produce tasks which are small and fragmented, the worker has no control over his/her work because the conception of the task has been separated from its execution. Braverman (1974) has argued that there has been a general tendency to de-skill and routinize jobs across the employment spectrum. Taylorism can be seen where nurses are required to adhere to rigid procedures and routines and in the assumptions of 'manpower' planning in nursing.

In 1832 Charles Babbage had recognized the potential to weaken the bargaining power of workers by fragmenting work tasks. Taylor took this a step further, believing that it was possible to treat each worker as an individual economic unit. Taylor wanted a different rate for every worker in order to eliminate any 'community of interest' between workers. We can rediscover his influence in the recent moves away from collective bargaining and in favour of performance-related pay.

Fordism

Taylorism coincided with the development of the moving assembly line and that system of production that has come to be known as Fordism. Henry Ford apparently adopted the moving assembly line after watching workers in his local abattoir in the process of disassembling cattle. Fordism combined Taylorist management practices with the intensification of production through increased automation. The goal of Fordism was the large-scale mass production of goods in order to achieve economies of scale. Fordism also recognized that mass-produced goods required mass markets. The higher wages offered to workers as an incentive to work in the car industry were also a recognition that factory workers were to become important consumers of mass-produced goods (Watson 1987). The rise of Fordism has been linked to the growth of the welfare state with its need to promote stable markets for mass-produced goods by ameliorating the economic consequences of personal misfortunes such as unemployment and ill-health.

Recent commentators have suggested that we are moving into a post-Fordist era. Changes in work, employment and the welfare state have been attributed to this transition. In addition, it has been suggested that with the decline in large-scale manufacturing, we have moved to a post-industrial society, a society in which different skills are required of the workforce.

A service society?

Bell (1973) among others has described contemporary society as 'post industrial'. Bell presents a benign vision of a society in which the majority work in personal service industries and 'dirty' jobs like mining become a thing of the past.

In the post-war period there has been a marked changed in the economic structure of the UK and thus a change in employment patterns. Manufacturing industries such as steel and shipbuilding have declined, leading to large-scale unemployment in areas such as the North East of England and South Wales. This has been in part due to the creation of 'global' markets leading multinational companies to move labour-intensive industries to countries where labour costs are cheaper, such as South East Asia. At the same time automation and the growth of information technology have allowed industries to shed workers in a process of 'industrial shakeout' encouraged particularly through the 1980s to increase efficiency and competitiveness.

During this period the service (or tertiary) sector has increased in size and importance with the growth of services such as banking, retailing, leisure industries and to some extent health care. The growth in the size and importance of the service sector has been referred to as the 'tertiarization' of the economy and it has a number of implications. First, it implies a growth in white collar jobs and a corresponding decline in manual work. Second, jobs in service industries such as shop work and office work employ a different set of skills. Physical skills become less important than interpersonal skills. Thus the growth in service industries had produced a corresponding increase in job opportunities for women and is in part responsible for their increased participation in the labour market. It has to be noted however that much of this growth of employment has been part time and low paid. In 1977 women earned 75% of male hourly earnings and by 1986 this figure had declined slightly to 74.3% (Walby 1989). There are implications for nursing because women now have greater choice of employment and recruitment and retention problems in nursing have led to attempts to recruit nurses from a wider range of backgrounds (Mackay 1989).

Emotion work

The growth in personal service industries has led to a growing interest in the different set of skills which such industries require. Hochschild (1983) has described the interpersonal aspects of service work as 'emotional labour'. Emotional labour involves work activity in which the worker is required to display particular emotions in the course of providing a service. It is a concept which has been rapidly appropriated by nurses to describe important aspects of their work. The appropriation of this term by nurses reflects the nursing project to reconstruct its identity around nurses' relationships to individual patients (James 1992; Smith 1992).

Most nursing writing on emotional labour has done little more than describe the emotion work of nurses and assert its importance. This is a pity as it ignores the central thrust of Hochschild's work which is to explore the management of emotions in commercial organizations. What is interesting about emotional labour is that it is managed and Hochschild is concerned with the array of management practices which have arisen to ensure that the workers' emotions are appropriated to the needs of the organization.

In Hochschild's study, Delta airline hostesses were exhorted not only to smile but to 'really mean it'. Hochschild employs a distinction between deep and surface acting to describe what is expected when emotional labour is required. In surface acting we try to change our outward appearance and gestures, tone of voice, etc. The other way is deep acting as propounded by the Russian director Constantia Stanislavski. Stanislavski encouraged actors to conjure up the appropriate feelings by training their imagination; to get into the shoes of the character. Airline hostesses were required not merely to smile but to work on their inner feelings in order to summon 'genuine' friendly and sympathetic service for the customer.

Managers do not always want to encourage a positive affect in their employees. Hochschild's study also encompassed the rather different emotional repertoire of Delta's debt collectors:

> The corporate world has a toe and a heel, and each performs a different function; one delivers a service, the other collects payment for it. When an organisation seeks to create demand for a service and then deliver it, it uses the smile and the soft questioning voice. Behind this delivery display, the organisation's worker is

asked to feel sympathy, trust and good will. On the other hand, when the organisation seeks to collect money for what it has sold, its workers may be asked to use a grimace and the raised voice of command. Behind this collection display the worker is asked to feel distrust and sometimes positive bad will.

(Hochschild 1983, p.137)

The emotions we feel at work have come to be subject to the control and scrutiny of managers. To some extent this marks the extension of Taylorist management practices to new areas of work. Sometimes this can involve the management of surface acting. The scripted interactions of the staff of fast food chains who tell us to 'have a nice day' come into this category. In service industries where interaction with the customer is more prolonged however management must achieve a more penetrating control of workers' emotions.

We might want to ask what relevance Hochschild's work has to nursing. If nurses carry out emotion work with patients surely this is because they want to. Most nurses emphasize the subjective and caring aspects of nursing as one of the reasons they chose nursing as a career. Airline stewardesses also entered their jobs because they wanted to meet and to help people, so where is the problem? For Hochschild the problem lies in the ownership of emotions. In Marxist terms emotional labour is alienated labour, it is labour which is no longer under the control of the worker. Hochschild quotes a section from 'Das Kapital' in which Marx discusses the testimony of the mother of a child labourer:

When he was seven years old I used to carry him on my back to and fro through the snow, and he used to work sixteen hours a day . . . I have often knelt down to feed him as he stood by the machine as he could not leave it or stop.

(Marx 1977 p.356)

The child described by Marx is an 'instrument of labour', his time, physical health and strength are appropriated to make profits for the factory owner. Even though it is a smile or a feeling which is now appropriated the emotional labour of the airline stewardess is appropriated to serve the needs of the airline company just as the mill owner appropriated the physical labour of the child described by Marx. The airline stewardess must smile at the most abusive and offensive passenger because the customer is always right. She must smile whether she wants to or not because the company has paid for her smile.

Hochschild considers the effects of industry speed up on emotion work. Increased competition in the airline industry led to increased workloads and throughput of passengers. Airlines continued to press for 'genuinely friendly' service while the conveyor belt got faster and faster. Queues were longer, breakdowns more frequent, complaints multiplied. Stewardesses and passengers alike found the system stressful, passengers could take out their frustration on the front-line staff but the stewardesses had to keep on smiling.

If the new managerialism in health care has brought us increased 'consumerism' it has also intensified the pace of work in the name of 'efficiency'. It has also brought stress and 'burnout' as we try to resolve the dissonance between holism and 'cost-effective' care (Wigens 1997). We need to ask ourselves not just whether nursing involves emotional labour but also who controls it and who benefits from it. To answer these questions we need to further consider recent managerial changes in health care.

Post Fordism and the flexibility offensive

If Fordism is typified by large-scale, inflexible production of standardized products then post Fordism is defined in opposition to this. A post-Fordist economy is characterized by small-scale flexible production made possible by the development of information technology. These technological developments permit the development of customized and specialized goods, fuelling a demand for products which project the lifestyle and taste of the purchaser. Designer label clothing replaces the standardized Ford car as a symbol of affluence and achievement.

Post-Fordist production demands a different style of work organization. Workers require greater skill and they must be adaptable and willing to acquire new skills and knowledge. They must learn to handle greater responsibility and in return are granted greater autonomy. Production is decentralized and hierarchies flattened.

Handy (1989) argues that the organization of the future is the 'shamrock' organization. One leaf of the shamrock is the 'core' professional staff whose knowledge is essential to the organization. The second leaf of the shamrock is 'non-core' functions such as catering and cleaning. This work is shed to outside contractors who, it is argued, will do the job better for least cost. These ideas were incorporated into the NHS with the introduction of compulsory competitive tendering. Commentators have questioned the contention that contracting out can reduce cost (Ranade 1994) and it is perhaps an irony given the legacy of Nightingale that cleanliness in hospital should be regarded as a 'non-core' activity. Finally, at the 'periphery' is a flexible workforce of less skilled workers employed as part-timers, temporary staff or homeworkers to accommodate peaks and troughs in demand and thus reduce the labour costs of the organization.

Some writers have criticized theories of post Fordism for their technological determinism. There is little evidence in the UK that changes in the workplace have resulted from modernized techniques of production. Instead the flexibility offensive is seen as managerially and politically driven, particularly through the New Right ideologies of the 1980s (Rustin 1989). State-run services have become experimental testing grounds for these new employment practices including the NHS reforms which culminated in the 1989 white paper 'Working for Patients'.

There are a number of changes in employment practice encompassed under the rubric of increased 'flexibility'. First, contract flexibility has entailed a move away from permanent to short-term contracts and the use of bank and agency staff. This implies the casualization of the workforce. Buchan (1994) found a marked increase in the use of temporary contracts in some trusts. Seccombe, Patch and Stock (1994) found a clear increase in the use of short-term contracts of less than one year in the employment of newly qualified nurses. Time flexibility involves changing working patterns to accommodate peaks and troughs and demand and reduce labour costs. Experimentation with rostering systems and a reduction of shift overlaps are occurring with an increase in 12-hour shiftworking (Buchan 1994). Skills based flexibility involves a move to 'multi-skilling' and an attempt to ensure that economies are realized by transferring skills to lower grade and hence cheaper staff, for example the transfer of junior doctors' work to nurses. Pay flexibility is introduced through local pay bargaining and the introduction of performance-related pay (Walby and Greenwell 1994).

Davies (1990) presented an optimistic vision of increased flexibility in which our new 'flexi lives' give us more leisure and the freedom to develop new skills and talents. Her work which laid the groundwork for the post-registration education and practice (PREP) reforms of post-registration education placed a new responsibility on individual nurses for their education and training through the professional portfolio. It optimistically views the nurse as steering her own career by a process of continuous improvement and self development. The shifting of the costs of training from employer to employee are seen as inevitable.

Much depends on whether nursing is seen as at the 'core' or the 'periphery' of the 'business' of health care. Nurses could be seen as a highly skilled and knowledgeable group in whom the service need to invest or an easily replaceable pool of cheap labour. Nursing may be restructured with a small elite of highly trained nurses controlling a large workforce of lesser trained staff. The introduction of nursing aides and recent changes in skill mix suggest this last scenario (Edwards, 1997).

The move to increased labour flexibility in nursing has occurred at the same time as nurses have been pursuing a strategy of professionalization, with the introduction of educational reforms and new methods of work organization such as primary nursing. Yet if nurses have been powerless to resist the casualization of the nursing workforce and the introduction of skill mix reviews which have led to a reduction in trained nursing staff, how successful has the professionalizing project been? Recent changes in health care have had contradictory implications for nurses and these reflect competing trends in the workplace generally.

Deskilling or professionalization? Post Fordism or McDonaldization?

There are two visions of the future and the present. One conjures up a world of work in which we are all progressively deskilled as managerial controls tighten and more of our work becomes prescribed and routinized (Braverman 1974). The other envisions the creation of a post-industrial knowledge-based society in which many more people will have rewarding jobs in the information and service sectors. A large 'core' of highly trained staff will be valued for their knowledge and skills.

Ritzer (1996) has argued that far from entering an era of post Fordism, we are entering an age of 'McDonaldization'. McDonaldism has extended assembly line techniques to the service sector. McDonalds is the success story of our time emulated by countless corporations both public and private. McDonaldism has four basic dimensions: efficiency (cost cutting), calculability (quantification), predictability and increased control through the substitution of non-human for human technology (robots, computer programs). As with all rationalized systems McDonaldization produces negative by-products such as the dehumanization of customers and employees and unintended inefficiency and waste.

As a counter to the argument that post Fordism has led to a breakdown of Fordist and Taylorist regimes of work, Ritzer is arguing that such regimes have extended enormously. For Ritzer the idea that we have entered an era of consumer choice and flexibility is an illusion:

> First homogenous products dominate a McDonaldised world. The Big Mac, The Egg McMuffin and Chicken McNuggets are identical from one time and place to another. Second, technologies such as Burger King's conveyor system, as well as the french fry and soft drinks machines throughout the fast food industry are as rigid as many of the technologies of Henry Ford's assembly line system. Further, the work routines in the fast food restaurant are highly standardised. Even what the workers say to customers is routinised. The jobs in a fast food restaurant are deskilled; they take little or no ability. The workers are homogenous and the actions of the customers are homogenised by the demands of the fast food restaurant (for example, don't dare ask for a rare burger).
>
> The workers at fast food restaurants are interchangeable. Finally, what is consumed is homogenised by McDonaldisation. Thus in these and other ways Fordism is alive and well in the world although it has been transformed into McDonaldism'.
>
> (Ritzer 1996, p.152)

McDonaldization has entered health care with increased managerialism. Managers have sought to increase predictability and control by increased surveillance of medical and nursing work. This has led to the introduction of clinical protocols and quality assurance procedures. Increased calculability is pursued through audit, performance indicators and the outcomes movement. The intensification of work achieves efficiency savings, for example by the introduction of assembly line techniques to day surgery (Wigens 1997).

In a prescient article Fourcher and Howard (1981) argued that nursing was torn between a 'personal rationality' in which work is organized in a unique and creative way by the individual worker and an 'organizational rationality' in which work is organized to suit the systemic requirements of a large organization. Nurses have aspired to the relative autonomy of the professions and have sought to imbue their work with a personal rationality of care. Primary nursing has been seen as a vehicle to establish autonomy in nursing. Primary nursing is seen to imply a decentralization of controls and a reintegration of the nursing role around a total relationship with the patient. Accountability and responsibility for individual patients provides a coherent focus for the 'new' nursing.

Ironically primary nursing may offer greater scope for managerial control of nursing. The rhetoric of decentralization in the healthcare reforms masked an increase in central direction of the NHS (Ranade 1994). At all levels of the NHS responsibility has been devolved downwards while power has been centralized. Devolved budgets mean that individual ward sisters are responsible for expenditure over which they have no overall control. An increased emphasis on accountability means that clinicians are increasingly held responsible for failures in the service. A new climate of risk persuades frontline health care summed up in the statement that nurses are constantly 'watching their backs' (Annandale 1996). Primary nursing has enhanced nurses' sense of responsibility but has not freed nurses from the rationalizing and cost-cutting imperatives of the organization. An increased sense of accountability may become a burden rather than an opportunity.

What price professionalism?

Many nurses have hoped that professionalization would improve the position of nursing, others have been more sceptical. A common approach to professions has been the 'trait' approach in which occupations seek to identify the attributes of a profession and ensure that their occupation possesses them. Thus nurses have identified a need for self-regulation, enhanced educational preparation and an esoteric body of knowledge. Wilensky (1964) suggests that more and more occupations are acquiring these traits so they may no longer offer the promise of advancement, merely the necessary conditions to preserve the status quo.

The neo-Weberian perspective on professionalization argues that professionals gain their status and power from their ability to achieve 'occupational closure'. Traditional professions such as law and medicine secured a legal monopoly over their practice and the ability to restrict entry. They also secured the ability to define the boundaries of subordinate occupations such as nursing.

According to Freidson (1975):

> By the turn of the century nursing had become a full-fledged occupation rather than a sideline of gentility or charity, and a fairly dignified occupation with a status independent of the clientele it served. As first established its "code" stressed skillful and intelligent execution of the doctors orders but in time the question began to be raised: "Are we still subservient or do we make intelligent responses to instructions?" The leaders of nursing came to be concerned that nursing be neither a dilution of medicine or an accretion of the functions medicine has sloughed off. While nursing originally established itself as a full-fledged occupation of some dignity by tying itself to the coat tails of medicine, it has come to be greatly concerned with finding a new independent position in the division of labour. (1975, p.63)

For Freidson nurses cannot fail to be subordinate so long as their work remains connected to medicine. Nurses are unable to control the boundaries of their work. Routine 'caring' work which they may value can be handed over to untrained or unpaid staff to cut costs. At the same time, nurses may be required to take over functions such as intravenous cannulation which medicine has 'sloughed off'. Conversely, where nurses' labour is readily available they may be required to take on domestic and clerical functions which could otherwise be performed by untrained staff. Witz (1992) has pointed out that nurses' subordination to doctors is not just a reflection of their place in the occupational order, it is also a reflection of the place of women's work in a patriarchal society.

The predicament for nursing lies in the fact that nursing has attempted to develop a personal rationality of care through narratives of 'holism' based around the 'lived experience' of patients (see Chapter 7). While nurses have constructed their account of their professional 'difference' around this narrative, it remains true that caring is still perceived as women's work and is undervalued.

Do nurses continue to assert the value of what they do or do they seek advancement by espousing other values? Nursing can still seek professional advancement on medicine's coat tails by taking on roles that medicine has sloughed off, such as the surgeon's assistant. Alternatively nurses can seek advancement by adopting the technical rationality of heathcare management and climbing the managerial ladder. What is the future of these varied strategies for nurses?

Nurses' subordination to medicine must be placed in a context of greater bureacratic–professional conflict. Flynn (1992) has argued that the creation of a more centralized bureaucracy and assertive management style has shifted control away from professionals, although frontiers of control remain unstable. A central theme of conflicts between managers and professionals has been the argument about who has the best right to represent the consumer. This argument has been pursued particularly through conflicting representations of quality. According to Clarke and Newman (1997):

> Many professionals have seen quality as a site in which professional practices and values may be defended and where they may be able to reassert a claim to both represent and advance user interests. At the same time, quality is central to the managerialist agenda of disciplining professional autonomy in the search for greater organizational efficiency. (1997, p.119)

Many reforms introduced in the name of consumerism have enabled managers to take greater control of public sector organizations. Clarke and Newman see the 'Patients Charter' as, in reality, a charter for managers, because it allows managers to define standards for the whole organization and to scrutinise professional work in order to measure compliance with these standards. Managers set their own agenda for consulting the consumer and the managerial view of quality tends to emphasize quality initiatives that can be achieved at nil cost (Cooke 1994). In contrast to the managerial view, professional constructions of quality emphasize the clinician's closeness to the patient and their expertise in meeting individual patient's unique needs.

While doctors have been largely successful in protecting their professional view of quality, nurses have been particularly vulnerable to managerial incursions into professional territory. A good example is the introduction of audit. While medical audit has remained a strictly confidential system of peer review, nursing audit has been transparent to management and has quickly been linked to workload studies aimed at reducing the cost of the nursing work force.

Clarke and Newman argue that conflicts about consumer represent-ation and quality represent political struggles between professions and managers about who has the right to control the high moral ground by claiming to represent the 'best interests of the patient'.

Managers and professionals may appear eager to co-opt consumer groups to their cause, but have little real interest in promoting the voice of the user within the organization. The politics of consumer representation is about control and autonomy at work and is often a political conflict in which the real user of the service remains a marginal figure. There have been some exceptions, such as the alliance between midwives and women's groups to promote the humanization of childbirth. It may be that the success of this movement relied on its ability to draw on the wider political movement of feminism.

As we have seen earlier, some contemporary commentators have argued that we are moving into a post-Fordist era in which skilled workers will have increased autonomy at work. Thus primary nursing has been heralded as an example of post Fordism in health care. Other authors have argued that Taylorist regimes of control have extended to new areas of work particularly with the new managerialism in public services. We can see these two processes as competing trends in the healthcare arena as we move, according to Jessop (1994), from 'flawed Fordism' to 'flawed post Fordism'.

Flynn (1992) suggests that we can look at labour process theory to explain bureaucratic professional conflict in health care. In 'high trust' systems employers are granted 'responsible autonomy' and are allowed to work with the minimum of supervision using their discretion. In 'low trust' systems where there are routinized tasks managers impose direct control by Taylorist principles.

In changing conditions there are shifts between these two forms of control. Control is precarious and is maintained and resisted through a series of moves and countermoves by managers and employees. At all stages the dynamics and outcome are shaped by group struggles.

Larson (1980) suggested that the fiscal crisis of the state has led to the need to rationalize the professional labour force, costs must be reduced and productivity increased. Flynn (1992) suggests that three strategies are used to achieve this:

> First a more fragmented and rigid division of labour, with greater specialisation and delegation of tasks to lower level workers; second, the intensification of labour, speeding up production, involving heavier workloads. Third routinisation and codification of high level tasks to facilitate intervention by non-expert managers. (1992, p.42)

Flynn suggests that these are real tendencies in the contemporary management of health care. We come back to the question of whose interests they serve. Hochschild suggested that industry speed up served neither workers nor customers. Some nurses have argued for the need to forge alliances with patients to promote nursing's rationality of care (Porter 1994). The ability to co-opt the patient may be an important key to the success or failure of nursing's continuing struggle to control its destiny.

References

Annandale E. (1996) Working on the front line: risk culture and nursing in the new NHS. *Sociological Review* 44(3), 416–451.

Bell D. (1973) *The Coming of Post-Industrial Society: a venture in Social Forecasting*. New York, Basic Books.

Braverman H. (1974) *Labour and Monopoly Capital*. New York, Monthly Review Press.

Buchan J. (1994) *Further Flexing: NHS trusts and changing working patterns in NHS nursing*. London, Royal College of Nursing.

Clarke J. and Newman J. (1997) *The Managerial State*. Sage, London.

Clarke M. (1978) Getting through the work, in Dingwall R. and McIntosh J. (eds) *Readings in the Sociology of Nursing*. Edinburgh, Churchill Livingstone.

Cooke H. (1994) The role of the patient in standard setting. *British Journal of Nursing* 3(22), 1182–1188.

Davies C. (1990) *The Collapse of the Conventional Career: the future of work and its relevance for post registration education in nursing, midwifery and health visiting.* London, English National Board for Nursing, Midwifery and Health Visiting.

Dingwall R., Rafferty A. and Webster C. (1988) *An Introduction to the Social History of Nursing.* London, Routledge.

Edwards M. (1997) The nurses' aide: past and future necessity. *Journal of Advanced Nursing* 26, 237–245.

Flynn R. (1992) *Structures of Control in Health Management.* London, Routledge.

Fourcher L.A. and Howard M.A. (1981) Nursing and the 'managerial demiurge'. *Social Science and Medicine* 15, 299–306.

Freidson E. (1975) *Profession of Medicine.* New York, Dodd, Mead and Company.

Gerth H.H. and Wright Mills C. (1970) *From Max Weber.* Routledge and Kegan Paul, London.

Giddens A. (1997) *Sociology.* Cambridge, Polity Press.

Goffman E. (1968) *Asylums: essays of the social situation of mental patients.* Harmondsworth, Middlesex, Penguin.

Graham H. (1984) *Women, Health and the Family.* Brighton, Harvester Wheatsheaf.

The Guardian (1997) £739 – the hidden earning power in your home that gets swept under the carpet. 7th September.

Hammond J.L. and Hammond B. (1949) *The Town Labourer (1760–1832),* Volume I. London, British Publishers Guild.

Handy C. (1989) *The Age of Unreason.* London, Business Books.

Herzfeld M. (1992) *The Social Production of Indifference: exploring the symbolic roots of western bureaucracy.* Chicago, University of Chicago Press.

Hochschild A. (1983) *The Managed Heart: commercialisation of human feeling*. Berkeley, University of California Press.

James N. (1992) Emotional labour, skills and work in the social regulation of feeling. *Sociological Review* 37(1), 15–42.

Jessop B. (1994) The transition to post-Fordism and the schumpeterian workfare state, in Burrows R. and Loader B. (eds) *Towards a post-Fordist Welfare State?* London, Routledge.

Larson M. (1980) Proletarianisation and educated labour. *Theory and Society* 9, 131–175.

Mackay L. (1989) *Nursing a Problem*. Buckingham, Open University Press.

Mackay L. (1993) *Conflicts in Care: medicine and nursing*. London, Chapman and Hall.

Marx K. (1977) *Capital*, volume I. New York, Vintage Press.

Oakley A. (1976) *Housewife*. Harmondsworth, Middlesex, Penguin.

Porter S. (1994) New nursing: the road to freedom? *Journal of Advanced Nursing* 20, 269–274.

Ranade W. (1994) *A Future for the NHS? Health care in the 1990's*. London, Longman.

Ritzer G. (1996) *The McDonaldisation of Society*. Thousand Oaks, California, Pine Forge Press.

Rustin M. (1989) The politics of post-Fordism or the trouble with new times. *New Left Review* 21st July, 55–77.

Seccombe I., Patch A. and Stock J. (1994) *Workload, Pay and Morale of Qualified Nurses in 1994*. Brighton, Institute of Manpower Studies.

Smith P. (1992) *The Emotional Labour of Nursing*. London, Macmillan.

Taylor F.W. (1947) *Scientific Management*. New York, Harper and Row.

Thompson E.P. (1968) *The Making of the English Working Class*. Harmondsworth, Middlesex, Penguin.

Thompson P. and Machugh D. (1990) *Work Organisations, A Critical Introduction*. London, Macmillan.

Wadel C. (1979) The hidden work of everyday life, in Wallman S. (ed) *Social Anthropology of Work*. London, Academic.

Walby S. (1989) Flexibility and the changing sexual division of labour, in Wood S. (ed) *The Transformation of Work*. London, Routledge.

Walby S. and Greenwell J. (1994) *Medicine and Nursing: professions in a changing health service*. London, Sage.

Watson T. (1987) *Sociology, Work and Industry*. London, Routledge.

Wigens L. (1997) The conflict between 'new nursing' and 'scientific management' as perceived by surgical nurses. *Journal of Advanced Nursing* 25, 1116–1122.

Wilensky H. (1964) The professionalisation of everyone? *American Journal of Sociology* LXX, 137–158.

Witz A. (1992) *Professions and Patriarchy*. London, Routledge.

6

The Nurse and the Patient

Introduction

In Chapter 5 we discussed a series of questions about the nature of nursing as a profession, examined its formal structure and relationships with the State and other professions, and made some observations about the nature of nursing work. In this chapter, we wish to shift our attention towards the patient as the focus of nursing work and nursing knowledge. Our discussion falls into four main sections:

1. An examination of empirical studies of the nurse–patient relationship.
2. The rise of ideas about holistic practice in nursing, and the subsequent tension between the *body-as-object* and the *patient-as-person*.
3. The notion of care, and its impact on ideas about nursing practice.
4. The problem of professional power, and of professionals as agents of social control.

As we pursue these four topics, we will explore several key concepts in contemporary sociology.

Power: Power is more than the capacity to compel an individual or group to undertake a particular task. Some kinds of power are coercive, of course, but more importantly, power is also about convincing individuals and groups that some kinds of talk and behaviour are legitimate: that is, creating a consensus.

Discourse: The term discourse refers to the way in which individuals and professionals employ particular kinds of strategic language to characterize their activities. This language both creates and is created by the objects on which it focuses. Biomedical discourse, for example, privileges the pathological: when we situate our thinking in such terms we are forced to focus our attention on the diseased body.

Object and Subject: The patient (and the nurse) can be characterized in two quite distinctive ways. First, as an **object** of discourses and practices – that is as an impersonal 'thing'; and second as a **subject** – that is an individual who experiences the social world and interprets that experience.

Social constructionism: This refers to a body of social theory, rooted in two different sources. First, in the sociological theory of Berger and Luckmann (1967), who stress the role of subjects (and intersubjectivity) in constructing a picture of the social world that makes it possible for us to see it as a taken-for-granted place and to function effectively within it. Second, in the work of the French philosopher and historian, Michel Foucault, who has explored the ways in which knowledge about the self and about the world is the product of particular kinds of productive and creative processes, in which discourse plays a crucial role.

In this chapter we will explore these sets of ideas, and examine how nursing has come to see the patient in a radically different way to that which was prevalent 30 years ago. We will draw extensively on ideas about discourse and the social construction of the patient as we do so. In each of the chapters of this book we have introduced particular aspects of sociological theory, as a lens through which different aspects of the human condition can be examined. The work of Michel Foucault, which belongs to an analytical tradition which explores the 'social construction' of ideas and practices, is especially valuable here. Foucauldian perspectives have become increasingly influential in the sociology of health care and the professions in recent years, but radically differ from other perspectives discussed in this book. However, a theoretical perspective is just that: it is a vantage point for 'looking at' social structures and relationships in a way that helps us to understand the processes and practices that go on within them.

Research on nurse–patient relationships: the technocratic model

The discussion that follows has two objectives. The first of these is to provide an overview of research on nurse–patient interaction in Britain since the 1970s; the second is to ask some critical questions about why such a body of work has come into being, and why it has taken the form that it has. The past three decades have certainly seen an enormous proliferation of studies – from sociology, psychology and from nursing itself – that have explored in great depth the conduct of the nurse–patient relationship.

It is now well established that nurses see 'relationships' with patients as an important part of their experience of work and of the organization of care. The relationship between nurse and patient is the site, of course, of particular kinds of work; however, it also permits the attribution of meaning – both moral and practical – to the generality of nursing work, and for many nurses a 'good' relationship with the patient is an end in itself. It is important at this stage in our account to distinguish between 'relationship' as a durable set of meanings attributed to encounters between the nurse and patient, and 'interaction' as the precise form that these encounters take. We shall turn to the latter first.

Verbal and non-verbal interactions between nurses and patients have been subject to considerable attention. Good communications skills are increasingly demanded of nurses, and much research has focused on how 'communications' are undertaken, and what technical improvements can be made in nurses' performance in verbal interaction with patients. This can be seen to fall into three main types of approach: research which explores the **duration** of verbal interaction; studies which explore its **content**; and studies which examine how nurses **control** their interactions with patients. For example, in one of the most systematic and methodologically exacting studies of British nurses, Macleod Clark (1983, 1985) used video cameras and radiomicrophones to examine 310 bedside interactions between nurses and patients. She noted that such interactions were short (their median duration was 1.1 minutes), they were primarily focused on practical questions relating to the patient's physical care, and that they were primarily controlled by the nurse.

Macleod Clark described four main conversational tactics which were used by the nurse to control the duration and content of their conversations with patients:

1. Closed questions, which led to simple yes/no answers from the patient.
2. Leading questions, which limited the range of possible answers that the patient could provide.
3. A rapid succession of questions, which left the patient uncertain about what answer to give.
4. Direct statements, which reduced the patient's opportunity to respond in any way.

These tactics are not always inappropriate, for there are many reasons why nurses and patients interact, and not all of these demand conversation of great duration. However, studies like that conducted by Macleod Clark have been used to provide a foundation for individualized nursing care, in which the possibilities for communicative exchange between nurse and patient are enhanced. As new ways of organizing nursing care, such as the nursing process and primary nursing, have been introduced, and as nurse education has become oriented around models of patient care that have expanded the remit of nursing work, research on the precise form that verbal interaction takes between nurse and patient has become steadily more critical (May 1990). Moreover, research has begun to take as its focus the 'context' of nurse–patient interaction, and the meanings that are attributed to it by both parties, rather than attempting to measure it. Even so, the conduct of verbal interaction appears to remain consistent across different hospital settings.

Research which criticizes the limitations on nurses' verbal interaction with patients conventionally falls back on two explanations, and both of these are inherently defensive. The first relates to the way in which it is profoundly difficult to individualize care in environments where staff are constantly moving from patient to patient or where there is a rapid turnover of patients, and involves the notion of 'stereotyping'. For example, one commentator has suggested that:

> although nurses claim now to have been concerned with the whole patient, with developing nurse–patient relationships, with individual patient care in the past, and although the trend in the past few years has been towards the individualised, planned and documented care of the nursing process; there is much evidence to

> suggest that then, as well as now, nurses tend to deal with types of people, types of behaviour, and types of disease, rather than with individuals.
>
> (Davies, 1976, p.273)

There is certainly reliable evidence that certain clinical and social characteristics do play a major role in eliciting negative perceptions of patients: psychiatric disturbance and violence (Jeffrey 1979); disfigurement or incontinence (Simpson *et al.* 1979); chronic and long-term illness (Melia 1981), have all been cited as being a source of such stereotypes. The sources of these variant labels are complex and ambiguous, but the principal source of negative stereotyping consistently appears to be the extent to which individual patients legitimate the nurse's role and are compliant, or disrupt nursing work through non-compliance. For example: in Heyman and Shaw's (1984) study:

> 80% of bad relationships were described in terms (. . .) categorised as non-compliance, such as complaining, demanding, ingratiating and disobeying. (. . .) This is consistent with findings in other research that fear of breakdown of control is more salient for nurses in their relationship with patients. (1984, p.70)

Control is a key feature of the second conventional explanation for the limited duration and controlled content of nurse–patient interaction. This relies on an interlocking relationship between stress and anxiety, and workload. From the 1960s onwards, it was demonstrated that particular patterns of verbal interaction were related to anxiety avoidance (Menzies 1970). More recently, workload has become an important feature of debate about nursing, and as we observed in Chapter 5, as nursing work has come to include a significant element of management and organizational work (Davies 1995), as well as changes in practice itself (the rapid shift towards short hospital stays, consequent on NHS reforms, for example), the volume and complexity of nursing work has greatly increased.

Research which takes as its focus nurse–patient 'interaction' focuses primarily on communications between nurses and patients as a technical problem of practice. This is investigated in terms of the activities, attitudes and behaviours that contribute to nurses' effectiveness in providing a particular model of care. Such work has typically characterized such interactions as routinized and strictly controlled. It would be easy to infer from such work that much verbal interaction between nurses and patients is superficial; but sociological approaches to nursing research take a somewhat wider view, and seek to understand the social contexts (and social construction) not only of the immediate encounters between nurse and patient, but of the various factors that exert an influence on these. It is to this 'contextual' perspective that we will now turn.

The nurse–patient relationship and holistic care

In Chapter 5, we showed that the recent history of nursing has been marked by a shift from ideologies of vocational service, to the knowledge-based practices of a professionalizing organization. In the course of this shift not only has the ideological basis of nursing been subject to radical change, but also new kinds of knowledge about nursing practice have been constructed. Underpinning these shifts, however, has been a dilemma for professional elites, about precisely the direction that these new forms of professional knowledge should take. Katherine Gow (1982) saw this problem as being organized in terms of a dichotomy between:

> Professional identity based on the development of a distinctive body of knowledge and professional expertise from which equivalence as scientific colleagues to doctors could be constructed.

Or:

> Professional identity as expressive specialists, derived from a distinctive body of knowledge about psychosocial dynamics and skills in therapeutic relationships.

This is a good deal more than a conflict between art and science. It reflects a key historical transition in the way that nursing as a profession attributed an identity to the generality of its patients and a meaning to its work. For in the past 20 years nursing has increasingly come to make the claim that it seeks to care for the 'whole person': that is, the patient is more than an instance of disease or trauma to be treated (an 'object' of biomedical knowledge and practice), but has a 'lived experience' of ill-health that involves wider social and psychological factors, and in which the boundaries between objective pathology and subjective experience are deliberately blurred. Within such a model, pathology is only one part of a complex matrix (Porter 1997). In this context, individualized care comes into the foreground, and the nurse–patient relationship becomes a crucial therapeutic instrument.

Nursing work, then, is increasingly not only conceptualized as a set of knowledge-based practices directed at actual or latent instances of ill-health, but also as a set of activities that have a wider function in terms of the patient's psychological and social adjustment. Nevertheless, the shift towards 'relationships' as a therapeutic instrument brings in its wake a particular set of problems, and Bjork (1996) has set these out in relation to the apparent decline of interest amongst nursing researchers in bodily comfort and care. She argues that:

> reviewing research findings over a forty year span (. . .) patients have more or less maintained a stable perception that good nursing care reveals itself first of all through the practical, technical or manual aspects of physical care. Nurses have, after an initial agreement with patients also shown a stable view of what is the most important nursing behaviour (. . .) this is the psychosocial support of patients through interpersonal relations (1996, p.8).

There is an apparent dissonance, then, between the views of patients and of nursing elites. But something else is also going on in the transition to 'holistic' care. First of all, the shift to holism is part of an attempt by nursing to construct a more enlightened model of practice in which patients feel that they are not simply 'objects' of nursing work (May 1992; Porter 1997). Second, it is about packaging nursing work in a new way that helps the nurse make sense of the context in which she or he encounters the patient. The shift to holistic nursing involves the construction of discourses of professional identity – the development of a strategic language that defines what nursing work is, and what it means. We can see the relevance of this if we turn to an empirical study that explores the dimensions of the nurse–patient relationship as they are accounted for by nurses in practice.

Knowing the patient: an empirical study

Debate about the place of discourses of holism is important because it offers a point at which we can examine very broad issues relating to the organization of nursing as a profession, and ask questions about the relationship between nursing and its patients at a macro-level. Examining the interactions that take place between nurses and their patients at a micro-level, however, helps us to understand not simply how discourses of holism are used to 'package' nursing work, but also how this work is negotiated with patients and others. At this stage it is helpful to draw upon an empirical study conducted by one of us (May 1992) which explored the ways in which nurses conceptualized their interaction with patients on general medical and surgical wards. The central problem at which this study was directed was, what does it mean to 'know' the patient?

In this study, as in others (e.g. Macleod 1994), nurses' accounts of patient care were dominated by the importance of somehow knowing them as 'individuals' or as 'whole people'. Underpinning these practical accounts of nursing work is the notion, which as we have noted, circulates in the wider professional discourses of nursing, that the organization of healthcare services – especially in hospitals – actually reduces people to objects. That is they become 'things' defined by pathology rather than by their social and psychological characters. In this context, nurses' accounts of knowing their patients revolved around striking a balance between understanding the dimensions and implications of a particular disease state, and gathering knowledge about how the patient responded to being ill. That is, nurses were involved in organizing their knowledge about the practical aspects of physical care, and a wider approach to caring for the 'patient-as-person'. In the following extract from a tape-recorded interview a nurse describes why this kind of knowledge has an immediate relevance to her work:

CRM: So what kinds of information are you after?

Nurse: I suppose, basically, what they were like before they came into hospital, so that we can maintain as normal [a routine] as possible – I don't feel that by coming into hospital that an individual should change their life drastically. I try to work round patients a bit more. We have a man in just now who at home – he lives alone – he doesn't eat after 6 o'clock and he just has tea and a sandwich then. And we just plonk down a three course meal at 6.30 and say "oh no, he's not eating". But the man doesn't eat at that time at home, he just *doesn't*. (. . .) it must be really abnormal coming into hospital in the first place, and I try to keep some sort of reality in their lives during their stay.

This kind of concern with the wider psychosocial aspects of the patient rather undercuts the radical critique of holistic nursing outlined by writers like Bjork (1996) that we noted earlier. It fits with nursing work precisely because of its practical value in organizing work that helps to make the patient comfortable. But more than this, it is intellectually and emotionally rewarding for the nurse and thus adds value to nursing work. We can see this very clearly in the following extract from an interview with another nurse:

> Because we do keep patients longer we do get more involved, you get more involved with families and with patients themselves and I find that quite rewarding. I like having a lot of contact with patients – and the setting they come from. You know, quite a lot of nurses set the nurse–patient relationship very much in the clinical area. I like to get the picture of what they've been like at home so that they *are* Mrs Jones or Mr Smith – you know – they're not the third bed on the left sort of thing. So I would say that it's an opportunity to have a good rapport with patients. And you're giving them a lot of back-up when they're coming in and going out – a lot of them with leukaemia need a lot of support.

This nurse gives an account of her work that shows how extending the provision of care beyond the operation of practical technical skills not only makes it more rewarding for her, but adds a value to it for the patient. However, we need to be clear that professional–patient relationships – at whatever level of analysis we choose to examine them – are not natural events that just happen. Instead, they are socially constructed. They are fabricated or manufactured through human agency, and within a context or structure that is defined by powerful social institutions. They reflect the existing dimensions of power relationships between individuals and groups: social class, gender, ethnicity and age; and they reflect the intimate relationship between power and knowledge. Similarly, they are subjected to powerful forces which exert pressures to change or transform the points of contact between the nurse and the patient, and which create conditions in which that point of contact is redefined.

Professional identity always exists in an uncomfortable tension with the practical exigencies of everyday work. The relationship between the rhetoric that surrounds interpersonal relationships, and the 'real' practices through which they are formulated on the ward is often difficult to apprehend. The sheer incivility of contemporary healthcare institutions, their industrial scale and complex division of labour, means that many of the interactions between individuals that take place within them are fragmented and episodic. Once again, if we look at an extract from an interview with an experienced staff nurse, we can see that this brings in its wake considerable problems and difficulties:

> Nurse: I think it must be incredibly frustrating for a patient to see so many faces. (. . .) I often feel – why should a patient give me their fears and worries, or make themselves vulnerable when they know perfectly well that they might not see me for another two or three days – or if they do see me I'm just passing through, because I'm not actually working in their area? In some ways it makes me reluctant to probe and to ask questions that a nurse should be asking – particularly of someone who's perhaps been diagnosed as having a terminal illness. What right have I got to expect them to make themselves vulnerable, when they're not going to see me again, or it's just going to be a very superficial contact? And I think patients are protective of themselves, and not unreasonably so.

Conversations are fleeting, and patients and staff may be constantly mobile within a built environment that is inhospitable to the conversations through which solid relationships are built. So it is important not to conflate relationships with friendships, for friendships are something quite different. These relationships may simulate some of the qualities of personal friendships, they seek intimacy, attempt to penetrate the private sphere of individual lives, and open windows onto occasionally awful and traumatic events. But they have boundaries that participants work hard to define and maintain, they may be uncomfortable and inhospitable and involve modes of behaviour that represent the exercise of considerable power.

While such relationships are organized in terms of core values and boundaries that are socially negotiated, they do also represent certain moral considerations. This is what sets them apart from many of the institutional relationships that exist between individuals and groups in other social domains, such as commerce or politics. There may be an urgency to personal contacts that is the result of physical or psychological incapacity on the part of one of the participants. Such relationships are organized through the fabrication of a social apparatus that is intended to meet the needs of those who by definition are unable to meet those needs themselves: they may mediate comfort for the sick and dying.

Power and control in the nurse–patient relationship

So far we have considered interaction between nurses and their patients in terms of a set of discourses about holistic care and professional identity. These sometimes seem to represent an idealistic and extensively moral picture of what nursing is, and what nursing work means. Within contemporary nursing, care and facilitation of the patient's return to health are vital components. However, the everyday business of nursing work is messy and contingent, and it relies on nurses being able to exercise power over their patients. In the final part of this chapter, we will turn to the question of power and control in some detail. In relation to the wide ranging psychosocial thrust of discourses about the patient-as-person, it is useful to reflect on Gerhardt's (1989) assertion that:

> Now the patient comes to matter as one who feels pain, or experiences satisfaction; that is, as the person in his or her entirety of previously clinically irrelevant identity. Through this incorporation of person-related aspects (. . .) the realm of what comes under medical control is broadened considerably (1989, p.325).

Throughout this chapter we have stressed the ways in which the professional discourses of nursing attribute an identity to the patient that is primarily located in the realm of the psychosocial. But this is a problem, since however much nursing work is identified in these terms, it is the healthy or unhealthy **body** that remains the central locus of nursing work. Nurses mobilize clinical knowledge that derives from biomedicine, to perform wound care or administer drugs; or to prepare a patient for an operation or deal with the aftermath of a stroke. At the same time, nurses manage the environment in which the patient is housed; they organize the ward, make arrangements for patient care, and organize medical care too. So while the patient-as-person is prominent in occupational and organizational rhetoric about care, the practical negotiation of work makes this difficult to achieve.

For this reason, professional power needs to be seen in terms that reflect not only the power to define the patient's clinical identity, but also in terms of the nurse's capacity to secure patient compliance and to ensure that patients do not disrupt the smooth running of the ward or clinic. It is now well established that nurses have a repertoire of techniques by which they deal with 'awkward' or 'difficult' patients in ways that can be quite coercive (Kelly and May 1982); and that, moreover, their judgements about such patients often have little to do with the kinds of psychosocial rhetoric that we have already described. Instead, the extent to which patients get in the way of nursing work, or are overly demanding, or cause administrative problems through 'unnecessary' complaints have vital importance in an operational environment where workload is high, and uncertainty is often great.

In fact, the very low levels of operational control that nurses may sometimes have over the circumstances in which they work means that they have to exercise power over the patient in quite sophisticated ways. Here, the kind of productive power that nurses are able to exercise by building relationships with patients, and demonstrating different techniques that emphasize 'care', have more than a moral value. Beyond this, such techniques draw the patient into a set of social relationships with nurses that counter many of the possibilities for uncertainty and disruption that exist on the ward.

Now, the role that discourses of holism play here is more than reframing the nature of nursing. They are also involved in building a consensus with patients that enquiries about their psychosocial state are not only legitimate, but important, when it is not always clear that patients themselves are prepared to go along with this (May 1995; Bjork 1996). As Burr (1994) observes, drawing on the work of Foucault, in her splendidly clear account of the constructionist perspective:

> What it is possible for one person to do to another, under what rights and obligations, is given by the version of events currently taken as "knowledge". Therefore the power to act in particular ways, to claim resources, to control or be controlled depends on the "knowledges" currently prevailing (. . .). Foucault therefore sees power not as some form of possession, which some people have and others do not, but as an effect of discourse. To define the world in a way that allows you to do the things you want is to exercise power (. . .). For Foucault, knowledge is a power over others, the power to define others.
>
> (Burr 1994, p.64)

In the constructionist perspective, knowledge and power are inextricably linked, and they find their expression in discourses that characterize and inform social practices. As we have noted, discourse refers to the way in which we use linked sets of concepts that act as a 'coherent way of describing and categorising the social and physical worlds' (Lupton 1994, p.18). Most importantly, a discourse provides a way of speaking (or writing) that attributes an identity and a meaning – and a set of purposes, intentions and motives – to our activities in specific settings, that carries with it the force of an abstract set of ideas.

Discourses of holistic care have formed an important part of the reconstruction of professional power in a period when the health service has become increasingly informed by consumerism. As we suggested in Chapter 5, consumerism changes the identity of the patient, who is no longer conceived of as a passive recipient of care, but is now someone who is actively adjudicating about the quality of services. Dingwall, Rafferty and Webster (1988) have shown how this shift to individualized care brought in its wake new and specific problems: organizing work through devices like the nursing process meant that while nurses were able to engage in closer relationships with their patients – and thus meet their own demands for a style of work that was more meaningful and desirable (Melia 1981) – that their personal qualities as well as their technical expertise were opened up to managerial supervision. In this context, we meet with what Foucault (1982) has characterized as a key means of exercising power in modern societies, 'surveillance'.

For Foucault and those sociologists who have employed his work subsequently, the extent to which social actors are monitored by others, and thus modify their actions and affects, is a vital point at which the exercise of power can be understood. In this context, power need not be seen as necessarily coercive, but is productive – of attitudes and behaviours, and of ways of understanding these. At a very crude level, we can see evidence of this in the way in which the placing of roadside cameras has altered driver behaviour. We know we are being watched, and therefore we are more careful about breaking the speed limit. But in Foucauldian analyses, surveillance is a more sophisticated phenomenon. For how we feel about who we are, and how we apprehend our experiences of the social world are examined as well as what we do. This new modality of expressing what we might call 'pastoral power' is an important part of work in the new nursing: an interest in the psychosocial aspects of patienthood means that new kinds of enquiries have to be made of the patient. Anxieties, fears, wants and needs outside of the direct care of the body increasingly fall within the remit of nursing. So, within the practices that make up individualized nursing care, it is the patient as an experiencing subject as well as an object of clinical procedures, that is the focus of a therapeutic gaze from nursing.

References

Berger P. and Luckmann T. (1967) *The Social Construction of Reality*. Harmondsworth, Middlesex, Penguin.

Bjork I. (1996) Neglected conflicts in the discipline of nursing: perceptions of the importance and value of practical skill. *Journal of Advanced Nursing* 22, 6–12.

Burr V. (1994) *An Introduction to Social Constructionism*. London, Routledge.

Davies C. (1976) Experiences of control and dependency in work: the case of nurses. *Journal of Advanced Nursing* 1, 273–282.

Davies C. (1995) *The Gendered Predicament in Nursing*. Milton Keynes, Open University Press.

Dingwall R., Rafferty A. and Webster C. (1987) *An Introduction to the Social History of Nursing*. London, Routledge.

Foucault M. (1982) Afterword: the subject and power, in Dreyfus H. and Rabinow P. (eds) *Michel Foucault: beyond structuralism and hermaneutics*. Brighton, Harvester.

Gerhardt U. (1989) *Ideas About Illness: an intellectual and political history of medical sociology*. London, Macmillan.

Gow K. (1982) *How Nurses' Emotions Affect Patient Care*. New York, Springer Verlag.

Heyman R. and Shaw M. (1984) Looking at relationships in nursing, in Skevington S. (ed) *Understanding Nurses: the social psychology of nursing*. Chichester, John Wiley.

Jeffrey R. (1979) Normal rubbish: deviant patients in hospital casualty departments. *Sociology of Health and Illness* 1, 98–107.

Kelly M. and May D. (1982) Good and bad patients: a review of the literature and a theoretical critique. *Journal of Advanced Nursing* 7, 147–156.

Lupton D. (1994) *Medicine as Culture*. London, Sage.

Macleod M. (1994) On knowing the patient: experiences of nurses undertaking care, in Radley A. (ed) *Worlds of Illness: biographical and cultural perspectives on health and disease*. London, Routledge.

Macleod Clark J. (1983) Nurse–patient communication: an analysis of conversations from cancer wards, in Wilson-Barnett J. (ed) *Nursing Research: ten studies in patient care*. Chichester, John Wiley.

Macleod Clark J. (1985) The development of research into interpersonal skills in nursing, in Kagan C. (ed) *Interpersonal Skills in Nursing: research and applications*. London, Croon Helm.

May C. (1990) Research on nurse–patient relationships: problems of theory, problems of practice. *Journal of Advanced Nursing* 15, 307–315.

May C. (1992) Nursing work, nursing knowledge and the subjectification of the patient. *Sociology of Health and Illness* 14, 472–488.

May C. (1995) Patient autonomy and the politics of professional relationships. *Journal of Advanced Nursing* 21, 83–87.

Melia K. (1981) Student Nurses' Accounts of Their Work and Training. Unpublished PhD Thesis, University of Edinburgh.

Menzies I. (1970) *The Functioning of Social Systems as a Defence against Anxiety*. London, Tavistock Institute of Human Relations.

Porter S. (1997) The patient and power. *Health and Social Care in the Community* 5, 17–20.

Simpson I. *et al* (1979) *From Student to Nurse: a longitudinal study of socialization*. Cambridge, Cambridge University Press.

7

Lay and Professional Perspectives on Ill-health

Introduction

Throughout Chapter 6 we observed that the therapeutic 'gaze' in nursing has come to focus not just on the specific disease or pathology that the patient suffers, but to incorporate a much wider definition of both ill-health and patienthood. This chapter, and the one which follows, explore notions of health and ill-health from a sociological perspective. In some ways, sociology is uniquely well placed to explore the ideas and practices through which ill-health is defined in contemporary societies, and how the individuals, groups and institutions that form those societies come to respond to it.

In this chapter we take as our starting point Turner's assertion that health and ill-health are best seen, not as objective categories, but as 'fundamentally social states of affairs' (Turner 1995). We conceptualize the causes of disease and distress as existing 'in nature' (e.g. in the case of influenza infection); or in the interaction between humans and the 'environment' (e.g. in the case of exposure to toxic waste materials). However, they are understood, interpreted and acted upon through human agency and in the context of social relationships – for our very ideas about what ill-health is are the product of interactions that take place within those relationships. Ideas about illness, then, have extended social and historical contexts.

Lay and professional knowledge

Sociology seeks to understand these contexts, and the interactions and relationships that are their components, in a holistic way. This fits well with nursing's attempts to understand health and ill-health as the 'lived experiences' that are so central to nursing theories and models. Our objective in this chapter is to explore the bodies of ideas that circulate in contemporary western societies through which these lived experiences are framed and interpreted. We need to do so, not simply from the reductionist perspective of those biomedical sciences which focus on **disease** (as an objective definition of pathology); but also from the perspective of those who experience **illness** (as subjective categories that structure self-identity and social relationships). This distinction between professional knowledge drawn from the biosciences, and the everyday ideas and experiences of those who suffer, is central to much sociological writing about ill-health. But it is important **not** to set up this distinction through the kind of naive dichotomy between knowledge and beliefs like the one that we have set out below:

> **Professional knowledge:** which defines ill-health in terms of pathology, legitimizes that definition through the authority of scientific knowledge monopolized by a specific social institution (medicine); and acts upon it by virtue of access to privileged expertise in diagnosis and treatment.

> **Lay health beliefs:** that define ill-health in terms of personal or group experience, lack the authority of scientific knowledge and privileged institutions, and act upon ill-health according to uncoordinated ideas about treatment.

The distinction between authoritative 'knowledge' and folk 'beliefs' that runs through so much discussion about individuals' ideas about health is often invidious. In sociological terms it tells us far more about the power relations that exist between those groups that are able to exert authority over definitions of illness and those that cannot, than it does about the substantive content of the ideas that circulate within them. However neither professional, nor lay, ideas about illness are homogeneous – they are often bitterly contested across a variety of arenas. There is, for example, significant disagreement within the medical profession, and among sufferers and carers, about the causes and natural history of chronic fatigue syndrome (and even about whether there is any such thing); similarly, disagreement exists about the extent to which much chronic low back pain is a function of organic or psychological pathology; or whether schizophrenia results from genetic inheritance or from social trauma. Nor is lay health knowledge necessarily naive and unscientific, it is often founded on experience, and it often works. Helman (1978) has pointed to the ways in which lay knowledge about illness exists in complex interaction with biomedical knowledge, and to this we could add that lay ideas about illness increasingly draw upon the knowledge base on which 'alternative' or 'complementary' therapies are founded (Sharma 1992).

Lay and professional beliefs about ill-health ought properly to be seen, then, as bodies of knowledge that are in engagement with each other, than as absolutely distinct. In making this claim, we are not saying that these bodies are equally 'correct' in their attribution of cause to disease and illness, nor that they offer equally 'valid' ideas about natural history or treatment. What is important, as Williams and Popay (1994, p.122) observe, is that they focus on different things. The biosciences take as their focus the causes and trajectories of diseases: lay perspectives, however, 'attempt to make sense of the causes of disease in relation to their impact'. Indeed, Williams and Popay argue compellingly that lay ideas about illness:

1. do not simply mimic the supposedly more sophisticated understandings of medical science;
2. are logical and coherent, even where their contents are at variance with accepted medical science;
3. are biographical – they are narrative reconstructions of the relationship between disease and experience;
4. and, they are culturally framed within certain systems of belief and action.

The organization of knowledge about health and ill-health within a society is crucial, in this context, to understanding the ways in which individuals and groups construct their own experiences, and the attributions that they apply to others. Professional and lay perspectives on ill-health are profoundly affected by the social and historical contexts in which they are located, and incorporate political, moral and other ideas about what it means to be healthy. Lupton (1995) has observed that concerns about health approach the proportions of a social movement in western societies. We use the term 'healthy' to attribute qualities of social good to persons and things; health in this context is a fundamental underpinning of individualism and independence – founding qualities of an economic and political system that relies on personal moral responsibility for individual prosperity and self-actualization. She argues that:

Under the prevailing discourse of "healthism", the pursuit of health has become an end in itself, rather than a means to an end. "Healthism" insists that the maintenance of good health is the responsibility of the individual, or the idea of health as an enterprise (. . .). Healthism represents good health as personal rational choice, "a domain of individual appropriation" rather than a vagary of fate. (1995, p.70)

Through the operation of such discourses we are encouraged to, 'release the potential of health lying inside us' (1995, p.71). This has obvious parallels with the way in which we are encouraged to fulfil our potential in the economic sphere. To be healthy, then, is to fulfil moral and political requirements around self-realization, and to avoid dependence on the State or others. Health is thus a matter of normative moral conduct, in which we are required to conceive of ourselves in particular ways, and to behave accordingly. In consequence, disease and ill-health carry with them moral consequences, ideas about the boundaries between culpability and susceptibility, that we must negotiate when we are sick. The experience of ill-health is as Bury (1982) asserts, a 'biographical disruption' that forces us to reorganize our views, not only of our body or mind, but of our relationships with others.

The medicalization of everyday life

How has this social movement, characterized by Lupton (1995) as 'healthism', come about? One of the principal features of the development of biomedical knowledge has been the extent to which it has come to extend into virtually every corner of everyday life. In historical terms, practitioners of the biomedical sciences embarked at the beginning of the nineteenth century on a programme of research of breathtaking proportions. This involved in the first instance a fundamental shift in the way in which they approached the problem of disease. At the beginning of the nineteenth century, the medical view of disease was one that was, in many ways, very similar to the practical definition of illness that we have given above. It relied on the patient's account of her or his symptoms, and on cursory observations of the surface features of the disorder: the patient's description of symptoms; the appearance of the body; the colour of urine; and so forth. One author describes this model of practice thus:

> For physicians and sufferers alike, a sick person's condition was seen to follow from a combination of errors of various sorts, many of which were held to be the consequence of self neglect. Faults in constitution, inheritance, diet, bowel habits, sexual activities, exercise, sleeping patterns and so forth were described as combining to produce disease. Although this disease might have a name (. . .) what mattered were the symptoms peculiar to the sufferer and the unique disturbance of solids and fluids that produced them. The first of the physician's skills lay in reasoning out what this particular disturbance was, from his knowledge of the sufferer's life and the recent history of the sickness.
>
> (Lawrence 1994, p.11)

Contemporary medical practice is very different. The two intervening centuries have been characterized by advances in knowledge and practice on a remarkable scale. Subjective accounts of symptoms have given way to diagnoses of disease. As we have already noted, when we speak about **disease** we normally refer to a specific pathological entity that can be objectively defined and located through practices derived from the biomedical sciences. The past two centuries have seen enormous effort devoted to identifying diseases: understanding the means by which they may be identified (signs); their causal mechanisms (aetiology); their effects upon the person (natural history); and their distribution across populations (epidemiology). The discovery of disease itself takes two forms: the general identification of a pathological entity such as AIDS (discovery), through encountering and describing some unfamiliar effect upon the person or through observing changes in reported morbidity and mortality; and the application of this description to a particular individual or group (diagnosis). This enterprise has led to the construction of an enormous taxonomy of disease states, that is, of **potential diagnoses and treatments** that may be applied in particular cases.

As biomedical knowledge has grown, so too has the power and authority of those professional groups who possess this knowledge and the means of interpreting it, to those who require it. In Chapter 5, we have discussed some of the ways in which the ownership and control of such knowledge is regulated and legitimized through the

State, but it is vital to note that autonomous mastery of this knowledge by the health professions, and by the enterprises that serve them, brings with it enormous economic and political power.

Critiques of medicalization have taken as their focus the exercise of this power. Radical commentators such as Illich (1975) have seen its origins in the growth of institutions such as the medical profession, pharmaceutical industry and governments that can control definitions of health in ways that leave ordinary people dependent upon monopolies of knowledge and practice. Illich called this process 'iatrogenesis' and saw it taking three broad forms:

1. **Clinical iatrogenesis:** where individuals are persuaded to surrender control of themselves to individual institutions and practices that may do them harm. That is individual autonomy over definitions of health is lost to powerful social actors who decide their future health state, and who may conceal the uncertainty and ineffectiveness of the treatments that they offer: for example, in the domain of genetic testing.
2. **Social iatrogenesis:** where the expansion of the biosciences and their associated professions has led to dependence on them for definitions of the self, and passivity in the face of this process. For example, the medicalization of old age (Harding, in press).
3. **Structural iatrogenesis:** where the immense power of the biomedical sciences and their associated industries and bureaucracies has deprived individuals and groups of the capacity to understand, or cope, with their ill-health in any meaningful way. That is, lay people have lost the capacity to understand their health on any terrain other than that set out by the biosciences.

For critics like Illich, writing in response to the cultural and political shifts of the 1960s, the growth of medical knowledge and power was a component of the rise of industrial capitalism and the consequent loss of personal autonomy in the face of massive social institutions. Other writers have focused more purposefully on medical knowledge and power as a means of social control. Szaz (1971), for example, has forcefully argued that medical labels – attributions of social identity, as well as clinical diagnoses – are applied to individuals in ways that legitimize control over behaviours that are socially unacceptable. Persons with mental health problems, for example, can be contained within institutions against their will. Similarly, particular social groups can be pathologized by virtue of characteristics that the wider society defines as being in some way 'other', often for arbitrary reasons rather than because of the existence of 'real' pathology. Parker *et al.* (1995), for example, note that Black British people are more likely to be admitted to psychiatric care involuntarily than their white counterparts, and that women are more likely to receive psychiatric diagnoses than men.

The idea that medicalization is a means of exercising social control over individuals and groups has been primarily applied to problems around mental health, rather than organic disease, because what is at issue is behaviour that is in some way deviant from expectations of everyday normative conduct. Behaviours and thoughts that are in some way troublesome for elite groups in society can easily be redefined in pathological terms, according to social judgements. The attribution of a diagnosis of mental illness was commonly used in the post-Stalinist Soviet Union to incarcerate those who publicly disagreed with the political system in place there. Similarly, gay men have historically found themselves involuntarily diagnosed as suffering from a mental illness leading to sexual deviation, rather than being seen as having made choices about their sexual orientation. In Britain, large numbers of women who became pregnant while unmarried found themselves incarcerated in lunatic asylums in the first quarter of this century, while in the preceding century the proportion of Irish immigrants who were involuntarily admitted to such institutions due to insanity resulting from habitual drunkenness was much greater than that of their English counterparts (May 1997a). Monopoly expert control over the ways in which social behaviour can be defined as representing an underlying pathology is crucial to the process of medicalization. One commentator has noted that:

> By defining a problem as medical it is removed from the public realm where there can be discussion by ordinary people and put in a place where only medical people can discuss it (. . .). The increasing acceptance among the more educated segments of our populace, of technical solutions – solutions administered by disinterested politically and morally neutral experts – results in the withdrawal of more and more areas of human experience from the realm of public discussion. For when drunkenness, juvenile delinquency, sub par performance, and extreme political beliefs are seen as symptoms of an underlying illness or biological defect the merits of such behaviour or beliefs need not be evaluated.
>
> (Conrad, 1975, p.14)

Radical critiques of medicalization, however, neglect the extent to which medical definitions of social problems and personal distress are eagerly sought by much of the population. We live in an age of expertise, where scientific knowledge rather than moral knowledge (such as religion or philosophy) is conceptualized as the supreme arbiter of problems in public policy and private life (May 1997b). In this context, personal problems are easily converted into medical ones. The situation is paradoxical, as Lupton (1994a) asserts:

> Western societies (. . .) are characterised by people's increasing disillusionment with scientific medicine. Paradoxically, there is also an increasing dependence on biomedicine to provide answers to social as well as medical problems. (. . .) Medical views on health, illness, disease and the body dominate public and private discourse. (1994, p.1)

What Lupton is driving at here is that medical knowledge about the person has assumed the role of a secular belief system, that displaces moral considerations about conduct and behaviour, and which provides an opportunity to redefine the self in functional terms. The medicalization of alcohol misuse in the nineteenth century, for example, drew new domains of moral conduct into the realm of medical definition and arbitration, while absolving individuals of responsibility for themselves (May, 1997a). Similar considerations apply to the rapid development of ideas about 'conduct disorders' at the end of the twentieth century (Conrad 1975; Parker *et al.* 1995). The growth of ideas about 'genetic health' and of the science of clinical genetics offers an opportunity to redefine almost every aspect of human identity and behaviour in medical terms, as we shall shortly see.

Points of engagement and resistance with biomedicine: lay beliefs about health and treatment

Critics of medicalization as a social and political process have tended to portray biomedical knowledge and practice as somehow monolithic. In this book we take a rather different tack: although there is tremendous evidence – both historical and contemporary – for the extension of biomedical ideas about health into everyday life, we need also to see that there are points at which individuals and groups engage and resist it. Although professional definitions of what it means to be sick dominate particular institutional contexts, lay knowledge co-opts and harnesses these definitions, or actively works against them. So, when we come to consider lay health beliefs we need to do this in the context of their engagement with biomedicine. To do this is not to underplay the importance of lay beliefs or to see them as somehow subsidiary to medical knowledge, but rather to recognize that the sheer explanatory power of the latter exercises remarkable influence over the ways in which ordinary people conceptualize health and illness.

Studies of the ways in which everyday health beliefs structure ideas about illness causation go some way to confirming such a view. Chrisman (1977) identifies four broad categories of health beliefs:

1. **Invasion**: in which some external agent – such as a virus, bacteria or object – assaults the body. This broadly accords with biomedical notions of infection, and deploys a military metaphor. An example of this kind of model may be found in sociological studies of lay beliefs about HIV infection (see Lupton 1994b).
2. **Degeneration**: in which the body becomes physically worn out through the effects of gradual failure of the organs or through damaging effects of environmental toxins. Studies of a range of chronic illnesses have suggested such a model (e.g. Gerhardt (1996), study of people with end-stage renal failure).
3. **Mechanical**: where some damage or blockage takes place within the body preventing its effective functioning. Problems associated with sexual function and infertility are frequently conceptualized in such a way (see Brodsky 1995).
4. **Balance**: in which the interior harmony of body and mind breaks down in the face of poor diet, drug misuse or stress. Much of the language of health promotion stresses the importance of balance and moderation (Lupton 1995).

Perhaps these kinds of models are best described as lay views **about** medicine rather than lay health beliefs, for they exist in parallel to explanatory models mediated through the biosciences. What is important here, however, is the extent to which beliefs about ill-health and about risk are individualized. Blaxter's (1983) study of working-class women and Backett's (1992) study of middle-class families have both pointed to the ways in which these lay constructions involve little notion of the distribution of ill-health: instead they relate to individuals' constructs of the reasons for their own health status. Blaxter, for example, stresses ideas about the 'randomness' of some kinds of ill-health, and Morgan *et al.* (1985) comment that:

> [Blaxter] suggests that although the women's models of causal processes were often inaccurate from a scientific point of view, they were not in principal unscientific. She argues that not only are women's models of disease causation sophisticated but they in many ways parallel modern scientific explanations, especially those that link the environment and health. (1985, p.96)

Alternative belief systems, equally sophisticated in their form, may be found in studies which explore the lay knowledge of ethnic minority groups who engage their own 'traditional' health practices with those that are available to them through 'contemporary' health services. Thorogood (1993) has described the knowledge and practices of a group of older black women in London. She points to the ways in which they prioritize their beliefs and the use of traditional 'remedies' in ways that:

> act as a resource because they form a body of knowledge about the way that the body works and the sources of risks and dangers to it (symbolic and actual) which has grown out of the historical experience of these women. The way that they experience health and illness and the appropriate ways of dealing with this are an expression of their "culture", their history and their current experiences as black women. In this way, "culture" can be reappropriated and seen as part of a dynamic interactive experience. (. . .) home remedies are completely under the control of the women in my sample (. . .) and as such mediate their relationships with both health and illness (structurally experienced) and the institutional health care systems (1993, p.31).

Work which explores the ways in which ideas about health are culturally situated, such as Thorogood's, opens up a means of seeing health beliefs and practices as points of resistance as well as engagement. Defining health beliefs in terms of the absence of dominant patterns of secular scientific knowledge neglects the crucial links between ideas about health and other ideas through which self and group identities are defined. Chapple (1997), for example, has shown how lay constructions of menorrhagia among South Asian women in Britain involve the intimate weaving together of definitions of the body (as being 'cleaned' by menstruation); gender (what it is appropriate to discuss with male doctors); religion (the organization of ideas about the purity of women and the uncleanliness of menstruation in Islam), and fertility and motherhood (heavy menstrual blood loss is necessary to assist in subsequent conception). But although the women in Chapple's study organized their definitions of menorrhagia in these very specific terms, they also engaged with western secular models of menstrual function and ideas about what was 'normal' in terms of blood loss, and sought help when their blood loss exceeded this 'norm'.

The idea of 'traditional' health practices is equally important in secular western cultures, and we can see evidence of this in the rapid growth in popularity of alternative or complementary therapies (Sharma 1992). These too act as specific points of engagement and resistance to scientific medicine, stressing their historical antecedents and their contemporary differences. The principal difference that practitioners and users of such therapies stress is that they somehow attend to the 'whole' person in a way that the scientific reductionism of modern biomedicine cannot. Even so, some such therapies are closely tied to medicine in that they operate against the background of 'disease' models of pathology: homoeopathy, chiropractic and osteopathy are examples of such approaches. All have their origins in medical practice, indeed, all were invented by medical doctors. Moreover, some complementary therapies are available within National Health Service treatment programmes (May and Sirrur 1998). They should thus be understood as complementary therapies. Other such therapies – such as naturopathy or reflexology – actively stress their difference from modern medicine and explicitly set themselves up as alternatives to it. But what is distinctive about the users of complementary or alternative therapies, as Sharma (1992) notes, is that few of them do so on the basis of a complete rejection of scientific medicine. In fact, users of homoeopathy or chiropractic are likely to do so in parallel with orthodox treatments or at a point where (especially in the case of intractable musculoskeletal conditions or illnesses such as chronic fatigue syndrome) they feel that orthodox treatments have nothing left to offer them.

Resisting medical categories: the critique of biomedicine and the rise of the consumer

If lay health knowledge exists in parallel and close connection with knowledge drawn from scientific biomedicine most of the time, there are points at which individuals and groups actively resist it. We can find examples of this in the way that feminist critics of the medicalization of pregnancy and childbirth have worked to reshape ideas about how women should be cared for in these circumstances (Oakley 1984); in the rise of self-help groups and advocacy organizations (Kelleher 1994; Parker *et al.* 1995); and in policies intended to reconstitute the user of healthcare services as active consumers, rather than passive recipients of services.

The medical response to pregnancy and childbirth is a case in point. It has been marked by the rapid extension of medical knowledge and practice (Lawrence 1995). As Oakley (1984) argues, this has involved a shifting definition of pregnancy and childbirth from a natural process that is a normal part of the female lifecycle (but which for much of history has been marked by very high rates of morbidity and mortality for both infants and mothers) that was organized and managed by women themselves, to one where pregnancy is marked by potential pathology and childbirth treated as a medical event managed by men. Thus, the 'management' of pregnancy and childbirth involves medical 'treatment' in the form of analgesics and anaesthetics, as well as surgical interventions – in the form of episiotomies and caesarean sections – that are regulated according to the precepts of hospitals as institutions.

From the 1960s onwards feminist critics began to question the medicalized model of pregnancy. However, their focus was not on the process of medicalization in the abstract; instead, they pointed to the concrete ways in which the construction of pregnancy as a medical event served to disempower women, and to legitimize (patriarchal) medical dominance. Porter (1990) has shown how a combination of feminist critique and sociological research has served to shift both policy and practice in this sphere of health care. In a discussion of sociological studies of antenatal and obstetric care, she observed that:

research on women's experiences of reproductive health care suggested that the medicalization of reproduction was indeed experienced by some women as alienating, that some use of technology and intervention was seen as unnecessary, that there were tremendous problems in communications between women patients and their doctors, and that medical dominance over information and decision making in consultations was unsatisfactory for many women. (1990, p.186).

In this context, debates about the medicalization of antenatal care and childbirth ceased to be a 'simple' matter of contest over specific procedures and practices (such as shaving, induction or episiotomy); instead, the relationship between biomedicine and the pregnant woman became politicized in the most thoroughgoing way. 'Academic' research about the organization of obstetric care gave pregnant women a voice through which critiques of medical practice could be taken up by self-help and advocacy groups, such as the Natural Childbirth Trust and the Association for Improvements in Maternity Services. In parallel, considerable media attention became focused on the problem, commencing with a notable series of articles in the *Sunday Times* during the early and mid-1970s. Porter notes that the results of this groundswell of changing opinion at a 'consumer' level involved changes in professional practice, which have included 'increasing the involvement of midwives, taking antenatal care back to the community, and reducing the number of hospital visits' (1990, p.188). The medical profession itself has also devoted considerable efforts to improving the quality and depth of communication with patients. Most importantly, the political contests around the organization of antenatal care has led to significant shifts at a policy level, with the publication of the Department of Health's policy document *Changing Childbirth* in 1993.

Summary

In this chapter, we have aimed to show that ideas about health and illness are not simple or homogeneous, and nor are they directed at medically defined disease. Instead, lay and professional notions of ill-health exist in a complex relationship with each other. These relationships are – like other social relations – powerfully influenced by structural variables such as gender, class, ethnicity and age. Some commentators, such as Lupton (1994a), have argued that contemporary western societies are gripped by the paradox of high expectations of medical knowledge and practice, paralleled by increasing disillusionment with their effects. This is a real problem for the health professions in their responses to those in their care: much ill-health experienced by individuals who are involved in relationships with professionals is intractable and complex. It is often chronic, and thus not amenable to curative procedures and practices. Yet the biosciences offer a secular belief system, and thus place health and ill-health in a particular and vital relationship with the identities that individuals and groups attribute to themselves. This belief system parallels and informs traditional patterns of knowledge and practice.

References

Backett K. (1992) Taboos and excesses: lay health moralities in middle class families. *Sociology of Health and Illness* 14, 255–274.

Blaxter M. (1983) The cause of disease: women talking. *Social Science and Medicine* 17, 59–69.

Brodsky M. (1995) Testicular cancer survivors' impressions of the impact of the disease on their lives. *Qualitative Health Research* 5, 78–96.

Bury M. (1982) Chronic illness as biographical disruption. *Sociology of Health and Illness* 5, 168–195.

Chapple A. (1997) General Practitioners' Decisions on Menorrhagia and Women's Perceptions of its Treatment. Unpublished PhD Thesis, University of Manchester.

Chrisman N. (1977) The health-seeking process: an approach to the natural history of illness. *Culture, Medicine and Psychiatry* 1, 351–377.

Conrad P. (1975) The discovery of hyperkenisis: notes on the medicalization of deviant behaviour. *Social Problems* 23, 12–21.

Department of Health (1993) *Changing Childbirth*. London, HMSO.

Gerhardt U. (1996) Narratives of normality: end-stage renal-failure patients views of their transplant options, in Williams S. and Calnan M. (eds) *Modern Medicine: lay perspectives and experiences.* London, UCL Press.

Harding N. (in press) The social construction of old age as an illness. *Sociology.*

Helman C. (1978) Feed a cold, starve a fever: folk models of infection in an English suburban community and their relation to medical treatment. *Culture, Medicine and Society* 2, 107–137.

Illich I. (1975) *The Limits to Medicine.* London, Penguin.

Kelleher M. (1994) Self-help groups and their relationship to medicine, in Gabe J., Kelleher D. and Williams G. (eds) *Challenging Medicine.* London, Routledge.

Lawrence C. (1994) *Medicine in the Making of Modern Britain 1700–1920.* London, Routledge.

Lupton D. (1994a) *Medicine as Culture: illness, disease and the body in western societies.* London, Sage.

Lupton D. (1994b) *Moral Threats and Dangerous Desires: AIDS in the news media.* London, Taylor and Francis.

Lupton D. (1995) *The Imperative of Health.* London, Sage.

May C. (1997a) Habitual drunkards and the invention of alcoholism: susceptibility and culpability in nineteenth century medicine. *Addiction Research* 5, 196–187.

May C. (1997b) The moral ecology of research on the addictions. *Addiction Research* 5, i–iv

May C. and Sirrur D. (1998) Art, science and placebo: incorporating homeopathy in general practice. *Sociology of Health and Illness.* 20, 168–190.

Morgan M., Calnan M. and Mannin N. (1985) *Sociological Approaches to Health and Medicine.* London, Routledge.

Oakley A. (1984) *The Captured Womb.* Oxford, Basil Blackwell.

Parker I., Gercaga E., Harper D., McLaughlin T. and Stowell-Smith M. (1995) *Deconstructing Psychopathology*. London, Sage.

Porter M. (1990) Professional-client relationships and women's reproductive health care, in S. Cunningham-Burley and N. McKeganey (eds) *Readings in Medical Sociology*. London, Routledge.

Sharma U. (1992) *Complementary Medicine Today: practitioners and patients*. London, Routledge.

Szaz T. (1971) *The Manufacture of Madness*. London, Routledge, Kegan & Paul.

Thorogood N. (1993) Caribbean home remedies and their importance for black women's health in Britain, in Beattie A. *et al* (eds) *Health and Wellbeing: a reader*. Buckingham, Open University Press.

Turner B. S. (1995) *Medical Power and Social Knowledge*, 2nd edn. London, Sage.

Williams G. and Popay J. (1994) Lay knowledge and the privilege of experience, in Gabe J., Kelleher D. and Williams G. (eds) *Challenging Medicine*. London, Routledge.

8

Experiencing Ill-health

Introduction

In Chapter 7 we explored some of the ways in which ideas about ill-health are socially organized. Our emphasis was thus on the ways in which individuals and groups bring different kinds of knowledge into play when they think about their own health, and that of others. Studies of the social organization and construction of such knowledge involve, as we have seen, both macro-level accounts of the ways in which ideas about illness are represented at a societal level (e.g. Lupton 1995), as well as micro-oriented accounts that take as their focus the ideas that individuals and groups use to deal with everyday questions about health (e.g. Thorogood 1993). In this chapter, we are going to attend to the ways in which ill-health impacts on the lives of individuals and groups, and on their relations with others. At the outset, it is important to recognize that sociology deals with these questions in two quite distinct ways:

1. **Epidemiological approaches:** through studies of the 'objective' distribution of health-related problems, using quantitative data analysis. Here studies have shown how ill-health is unequally distributed among particular social groups; we have already noted that social class, gender, ethnicity and age are vital dimensions of this unequal distribution, and that this is reflected in data about morbidity and mortality.

2. **Phenomenological approaches:** through studies of the 'subjective' experience of health-related problems, using qualitative data analysis. Here studies have shown how different kinds of ill-health are interpreted and understood by individuals in their daily lives, and have brought into the foreground the ways in which they perceive the effects of ill-health on their identity and behaviour.

In this chapter, we will take as our main focus the latter approach to the study of ill-health. Social epidemiology is important, indeed it is vital to a proper assessment of the impact and effects of much disease; and quantitative approaches are often undervalued in contemporary social science. In taking the approach that we have in this chapter, however, we recognize the value of the position adopted by many qualitative researchers in stressing that to appreciate the nature of the experience of different kinds of ill-health we need to explore this from the subjective point of view of the sufferer. This view is set out neatly by Karp (1996) in his study of people with depression:

> The essential problem with nearly all studies of depression is that we hear the voices of a battalion of mental health experts (. . .) and never the voices of depressed people themselves. We do not hear what depression feels like, what it means to receive an official diagnosis, or what depressed people think of therapeutic experts. Nor do we learn the meanings that patients attach to taking psychotropic medications, whether they accept illness metaphors in assessing their condition (. . .) or how depression influences their occupational strategies and career aspirations (1996, pp.11–12).

Sociological studies of ill-health can perform precisely this task. In fact, with its battery of qualitative research techniques and bodies of theory in which these are located, sociology is uniquely well equipped to provide a perspective on what it **means** to be ill, and how experiences of illness are organized. Our objective in this chapter, then, is to not only provide a framework for considering the experience of illness, but also to convey some of our enthusiasm for explicitly sociological approaches to understanding these experiences. There is an extraordinarily abundant literature around what we can loosely call the phenomenology of ill-health, and it is thus impossible for us to review it systematically in this chapter. Instead, we will introduce some central concepts in the sociology of ill-health, and then discuss these in relation to particular kinds of conditions. In particular, we will explore:

1. **Self-identity:** that is, the ways in which individuals come to see themselves as particular kinds of social actors, and to attribute a variety of meanings to their definition of the self.
2. **Role:** in which individuals and groups come to act in ways that meet particular kinds of socially organized 'scripts' through which their identity and behaviour is made sensible to others.

3. **Career:** by which we mean the way in which a particular condition extends through the sufferer's biography, changing the course of their life and engendering new experiences of the self and others.
4. **Stigma:** where individuals and groups have to respond to external attributions of identity, and where these attributions confer on them identities that lead to negative effects in their everyday lives.

One way to put these apparently disparate concepts together is to place the experience of illness within a dramatic context. In his autobiography *The Last Enemy,* Richard Hillary (Hillary 1941) describes his experiences as a fighter pilot during the Battle of Britain. The book begins with some self-characterization, Hillary is a man in his early twenties, and like most young men describes himself as someone who enjoys life in a carefree way, he describes his interests and his friendships, and his training as a fighter pilot. Gradually he comes to characterize himself first and foremost as a fighter pilot: he identifies himself with a particular social group and takes on the patterns of talk and behaviour that act as internal (self-identity) and external (role) identifiers for that group.

In the summer of 1940 his aircraft was shot down over southern England, and Hillary was horribly disfigured by burns and other injuries. This brutally exemplifies the kind of biographical disruption that ill-health brings with it. Both literally and sociologically, Hillary's career changes course: he becomes defined not by his own self-identification as a fighter pilot, but rather by his experience of his own injuries, for he can no longer do the things that he used to do and still wishes to. Instead, he is dependent on others for the most basic functions of everyday life. He ceases to be an independent actor, and instead takes on a new role – that of a surgical patient in a pioneering burns unit – the trajectory (career) of his experience is governed by decisions made by others. When taken on outings from the hospital, he finds that people recoil in horror when faced with his appalling and disfiguring injuries. He is somehow different from them and they reject him in ways that are sometimes trivial, but often psychologically damaging (stigma). As a result he is tempted to hide himself away from the company of others. Ultimately, Hillary recovered his self-identity: plastic surgery ameliorated some of the worst effects of his burns; and he returned to flying Spitfires. Hillary's autobiography was published posthumously, for he was killed in action in 1941.

Richard Hillary's autobiography is not much read now, but in many ways his experience – packed into a few months – exemplifies that of others, who suffer in less heroic circumstances.

Identifying illness

At the outset, it is important to understand that there is infinite variation in our experiences of ill-health. Only a tiny proportion of experienced symptoms ever get so far as being defined formally as a disease through contact with the health professions. For the most part, in our everyday lives we suffer many minor illnesses, often of uncertain cause and short duration. Headaches, menstrual cramps, minor stomach upsets, colds and flu are regularly experienced as inconveniences rather than illness. Existing epidemiological data shows an enormous 'iceberg' of minor symptoms concealed within everyday life, for which attention is not sought, because those who suffer them do not define themselves as ill or sick. Mechanic (1968) has set out a range of factors that can be demonstrated to lead to a definition of illness and subsequent help-seeking:

1. The extent to which symptoms are visible and recognizable.
2. Their perceived seriousness.
3. The extent to which they impact on the sufferer's life.
4. Their perceived frequency and persistence.
5. The degree to which an individual can tolerate them.
6. Knowledge about what symptoms may mean.
7. Anxiety about their perceived seriousness.
8. Competing needs (it may be more important to go to work than to seek professional advice).
9. Competing explanations for the symptoms.
10. Availability of treatment and assistance

In this context, the extent to which these factors are given weight by individuals and by other members of the social networks of which they are part will be of crucial importance in assessing the extent to which experienced symptoms are serious or not. But it is important to note that the interaction between individuals and networks is complex, and depends too on ideas which circulate in the wider society in which they are, in turn, located. The period since the war has seen the periodic eruption of concern about specific health problems – ranging from skin cancer to flesh-eating bugs, by way of Mad cow disease and seasonal affective disorder – that are given prominence by the mass media and become quickly locked into popular consciousness. Individuals and the groups to which they belong are increasingly exposed to a mass of information about disease and disorder, and struggle to make sense of this in the face of their own experiences.

While much of our knowledge of disease arises from clinical investigation and epidemiological studies, the anthropologist Byron Good (1994) has observed that much of what we know about **illness** derives from the stories that sufferers tell us. Sociology, with its battery of qualitative research methods, is uniquely equipped to explore these stories, and much sociological research in the field of ill-health has done precisely this. For if, as we have already noted – following Turner (1995) – ill-health is a fundamentally **social** state of affairs, then it is negotiated as much in the moral sphere as in the sphere of clinical knowledge about the body. We can illustrate this with a case study that also illuminates some of the factors that Mechanic (1968) suggests are important features of the processes by which individuals come to see themselves as suffering some kind of ill-health.

Bob's story: organic symptoms and private morality

Bob is a 44-year-old British male. In 1990 he experienced the first symptoms of Peyronnie's disease, a deformity of the genitals of unknown cause in which a small fibrous plaque forms, usually in the shaft of the penis, causing it to twist and bend on erection. The presence of this plaque makes sexual activity difficult and painful, and the disease has important psychological sequelae, as well as presenting the possibility of impotence.

> It started quite suddenly, I think. I was 37 and I had just moved north and had quite good job. What I noticed at first was a dull sort of ache. Really I thought I had just been a bit over-active one night and pulled something. But then I noticed

that when I had an erection it wasn't straight anymore, it was like, twisted. Immediately it wasn't very noticeable, but after a while it was just very obvious. (. . .) the first thing was that I was very nervous, actually I was acutely anxious because I could feel a small hard lump forming about an inch from the base (. . .) when I had an erection it was pretty obvious and very painful (. . .) the main thing for me was that I thought it was cancer. So I was very anxious and I spent a long time just sort of looking at it and worrying but I didn't discuss it with anyone and I got pretty introspective (. . .) what was difficult for me was this feeling that it was cancer and going to get worse and that it was going to have to come off. I know a bit about cancer because I have worked in hospitals on and off for 20 years, and frankly the idea of disseminating tumours was not as horrible to me as having my penis cut off. Partly because there is this thing, you know, that it defines you as a man. After all, it does.

In Bob's account the emergence of a visible 'lump' signals the onset of great discomfort and anxiety. The symptoms take several forms: the lump itself (as a source of anxiety about malignant disease); deformation of the penis (as a source of sexual dysfunction); and anxiety about, literally, loss of manhood. Every aspect of the self is engaged in this account, and bodily and social identity are given equal priority. Williams and Popay (1995) have noted that the question 'why me?' is of direct relevance to issues around lay experiences of ill-health. They note, too, that these questions are rarely addressed in studies of disease – which emphasize pathological processes and organic causality, rather than individual explanations. In Bob's case, he was able to develop a compelling lay diagnosis. Although he was in a stable partnership, in the course of his work he had met someone else to whom he felt increasingly attracted: the guilt and unhappiness that he felt about this were, for him, a convincing explanation of why he was experiencing these symptoms:

Here I was on the verge of having an affair and suddenly my todger was completely twisted. Well, when I thought about it like that I had a flash of understanding, that's the best way I could put it. (. . .) I had read something in *The Guardian* newspaper about a Cancer Centre somewhere where they were saying that there's a strong psychological effect on breast cancer, and I thought "well, I've been really emotionally stressed and I've wanted adultery and not wanted it, and now my body's reacting. My body is dealing with the parts my conscience can't reach." Because there's no doubt in my mind, if that hadn't happened I would have had an affair and that would have been it.

Williams has noted that in accounting for our illnesses we often do so on moral terrain: we wonder whether we 'deserve' a disorder and are concerned about the relationship between culpability and susceptibility. The crisis over HIV and AIDS has been a key example of the way in which moral (often sexual) attitudes and behaviours have been linked to susceptibility to a disease (Lupton 1994a). But in Bob's account of his illness, disease itself offers an opportunity for moral redemption. When he consulted the doctor, and was assured that the disease was, in effect, randomly distributed across the male population and that there was no special reason for him to be afflicted with it, his own lay explanation remained infinitely more convincing to him than knowledge imparted with the authority of clinical science. His explanation had practical utility, because it offered reasons for both susceptibility and recovery.

Ill-health as a source of stigma

Bob's account of his experience of Peyronnie's disease has some important things to tell us not only about how ill-health involves us in what Bury (1982) has called 'biographical disruptions' that demand that we consider our own identities, but also about how we believe that others will view us. In the early 1960s, the American sociologist Erving Goffman developed a compelling analysis of the ways in which states of ill-health are intimately related to the identities that are attributed to individuals and groups (Goffman 1963). Goffman undertook pioneering work on the sociology of mental illness, and this continues to be powerfully relevant after nearly 40 years because of the strength of its theoretical underpinnings.

Throughout this century, sociologists have been concerned with the concept of **role**: the way that in specific circumstances we draw on socialized 'scripts' and rules to frame our behaviour and verbal interactions. That is, we behave according to specific sets of socially organized rules and norms that permit and legitimize particular behaviours and activities. In the case of ill-health, the American biologist and sociologist Talcott Parsons developed the notion of a 'sick role' during the 1940s (Parsons 1951). Parson's starting point was that being healthy could be understood to be a social norm. Goffman's work (1961, 1963) dissects how people respond to the normative judgements of others, through an analysis of the ways in which they deal with **stigma**: that is, those features of their disorder that are generative of negative evaluations by others. Typically, analyses of stigma have been focused on those diseases that are visible and in some way frightening to others. Mental illness (Goffman 1963), epilepsy (Scambler 1989), Parkinson's disease (Pinder 1993) and some genetic disorders (Chapple *et al*. 1995), among others, have been demonstrated to lead to such effects. Scambler's account of the experience of epilepsy offers an important and helpful approach to understanding stigma, that builds and elaborates on Goffman's germinal work. One of the subjects in his study describes the experience of being categorized by others as suffering from epilepsy thus:

> People are ignorant of epilepsy. I don't mean "ignorant" rudely: I mean they're ignorant of the word epilepsy. The word epilepsy is like cancer, (. . .) they hate the word and they don't understand what's behind it (. . .) If someone mentions the word epilepsy – and once or twice I've caught someone saying: "Oh, you know that person suffers from, you know, that thing, where they have those convulsions" – I have to defend myself saying: "Well, I have a friend . . ." I defend myself through an invisible friend, because I can't say to them: "Well, I have that", without knowing damn well that I'd get sacked, and that they'd give me a very, very smug excuse for it.
>
> (Cited in Scambler 1989, p.56)

In relation to this, Scambler sets out the distinction between 'enacted' and 'felt' stigma. The first of these refers to concrete instances where individuals are discriminated against because of the social and cultural unacceptability of the condition from which they suffer. Here, the social risk that attends the public admission of a diagnosis of epilepsy is encountered in the form of possible or actual rejection of the sufferer by others. Enacted stigma, Scambler notes, is rather less common in epilepsy than individual (and isolated) sufferers may believe: nevertheless, it is an important component of the experience of many conditions, such as HIV/AIDS. Felt stigma, on the other hand, refers to the sense of 'shame' that sufferers experience – not necessarily because they attribute any degree of moral culpability to their condition – but rather because of their sense of imperfection. It is also a recognition of the possibility of enacted stigma. Sufferers thus conceal their disorder as much as they can, and thus retain a 'normal' identity in the eyes of their peers. Another of Scambler's respondents attested that:

It used to annoy me terribly, the shame of it really. I was so ashamed, very much so (. . .). My mother didn't like it [epilepsy] either, and it's obviously rubbed off on me (. . .) I wanted desperately to be normal. I didn't want people to say: "Oh, see how she's an epileptic!" To me it was a terrible time, and I used to suffer a lot, worrying in case I did take one, a fit, with one of the boys. I felt I could never tell any of them, anyway.

(Cited in Scambler 1989, p.84)

For all of the respondents in Scambler's study, the diagnosis of epilepsy was experienced as the attribution of a special status, that of being in some sense a social liability. This promotes a policy of non-disclosure that works to both conceal the condition from others. It also serves to constantly reinforce the sufferer's own knowledge that he or she lies outside the social norm. Felt stigma, Scambler observes, is thus 'more disruptive of the lives of people with epilepsy than enacted stigma' (1989, p.57).

In the previous chapter, we noted the importance of critiques of medical labelling: where the attribution of a diagnostic label has the effect of changing an individual's social identity, in a way that damages their life-chances. The enacted and felt stigma that individuals in Scambler's study experienced is an extension of this across a societal range. It is important not to assume that individuals are passive in the face of such attributions, or that the latter are somehow immutable and unchanging. Organizations that once provided charitable services for people with learning difficulties, such as SCOPE, now provide advocacy services that are intended to promote the wider interests of those who they represent. Many groups respond to stigma through the formation of organizations that are directly intended to confront it through political means: the health crisis over HIV/AIDS led to the well-documented stigmatization of gay men who suffered from it (Shilts 1990). In the face of political **opposition** to research about the disease and its treatment in the USA, groups such as Gay Men's Health Crisis and Act Up acted as interest groups to contest the Reagan administration's reluctance to devote funds to seeking the cause of, and cure for, AIDS. Gay men were, however, already well organized politically: AIDS emerged at the end of the 1970s, as a risk not only for the health of individuals, but also as a threat to the emancipation of gay men as a social category. It permitted those groups who rejected the legitimacy of the liberation movement which had worked since the 1960s towards de-criminalizing and de-pathologizing gay and lesbian relationships, to reconstitute them, not simply as a moral category – but as a direct threat to the health of the wider communities in which they were set. Stigma associated with HIV/AIDS was immediately the focus of political responses from those who did, or could, suffer from it.

The 'sick role' and the legitimization of illness

So far, we have emphasized that the means by which ill-health is defined and organized are not necessarily in the realm of scientific knowledge about pathology. Complex social factors also come into play in the transition from 'health' to 'ill-health' and in the redefinition of individuals as being situated, in some way, as being different by virtue of their health status.

The question that followed from this was, how could individuals depart from that norm in an orderly way, and come to occupy what they conceive of as a socially 'deviant' state? Parsons set up the answer to this in terms of the pattern of meanings and behaviours that structured the interaction between the sick person and others. His notion of the sick role is organized around a set of rights and obligations – a set of exchanges – through which illness behaviour could be organized. We have set these out schematically below:

Right: to withdraw from everyday obligations and duties.	Obligation: to accept definition as a sick person and to work towards recovery.
Obligation: to seek and accept appropriate advice and assistance.	Right: exemption from responsibility for recovery.

At this stage, two important comments need to be made about this model of the sick role: first, it involves a very specific view of what ill-health is, and how it is to be legitimated; second, it is highly culturally specific and assumes that the sick person has a range of choices about how their behaviour and social relationships – with kin and health professionals – through which these choices may be mediated. In relation to this, Turner (1995, pp.38–39) has argued that:

> sickness could not be considered merely as an objective condition of the organism without some consideration of the individual in relation to the social system (. . .). To be sick required certain exemptions from social obligation and a motivation to accept a therapeutic regimen. It was for this reason that Parsons classified sickness as a form of deviant behaviour that required legitimization and social control. While the sick role legitimizes social deviance, it also requires an acceptance of a medical regimen. The sick role was therefore an important vehicle for social control, since the aim of the medical profession was to return the sick person to conventional social roles.

The sick role thus provides a pattern for a set of social relationships that mediate ideas about normal activity and behaviour. In particular, it assumes a medical definition of sickness. However, as we have already noted, only a tiny proportion of experienced symptoms lead to individuals seeking help from the health professions. As Turner (1995) notes, 'not all sick people are patients, and not all patients are sick people' (1995, pp.43). Importantly, the rather restrictive model that Parsons set out tells us a great deal about the possibilities for episodes of acute illness, but much less about the trajectory of chronic or degenerative ones. It is easy to apply the sick role as an analytical device to a person suffering from pneumonia or recovering from a heart attack, but much more difficult to do so where individuals are suffering from long-term, limiting disorders. In the case of the latter, the sufferer may not be absolved from their responsibilities and functional requirements.

Suzy's story: negotiating the sick role

Suzy is 39 and is married with six children. For a number of years she has suffered from chronic and profoundly disabling back pain. Like many people with this condition, she has undergone extensive investigations which have failed to reveal any underlying pathology. Nevertheless she experiences constant discomfort, and often very severe pain. In the absence of a causal diagnosis, she finds this difficult to explain to others. When asked whether this upset her, she said:

> It does sometimes. I think it's because when I say to the girls or to my husband or whoever, "my back's killing me today" – and I get sick and tired of hearing it

as well. I mean, it's not like your leg's hanging off or you're covered in blood or you've got stitches in your head. You know, it's nothing you can see. But having said that, when it's really bad I could tear my hair out with it. But it's nothing you can see, so people can't say, "oh, she's broken her leg" I suppose. (. . .) Because if you can't see it and you haven't experienced the pain, you've no idea what it's like. And I'm sure people must think, "oh God, here we go again".

Much ill-health is clearly unambiguous, and individuals present with symptoms that are associated with pathological signs. The latter may involve some negotiation, and they may raise questions about the threshold at which a symptom actually represents a disorder. When, for example, does 'feeling low' become depression (Lewis 1995); or heavy menstrual blood loss become menorrhagia (Chapple, Ling and May 1997)? But in Suzy's case the circumstances are ambiguous: she experiences severe pain, but in the absence of medical evidence about its cause, she constantly has to negotiate the reality of this pain with others. She can offer no proof of its existence, and she is thus unable to provide an explanation for her condition that is useful in dealing with the people she encounters in everyday life.

And I was striving for a diagnosis, not just for me but for everybody. People say to you, "well, what's the problem?" And so I have to turn round and say, "I don't know". It makes you feel stupid – I went through a stage where I thought that because they could not find out what was wrong with me they were telling me that there was nothing wrong. (. . .) Are they trying to tell me that I'm having everyone on here? Am I going round the twist? I mean, I know they think a lot of it is psychological.

The lay experience of ill-health, in this case, involves not only apprehending symptoms and their effects (pain and disability) but also negotiating medical knowledge. Suzy wants to present her disabling pain as something that is legitimate and warrantable. However, where signs and symptoms are less easily understood by others, this warrantability cannot be assumed, and individuals' definitions of themselves as unhealthy are often contested.

Modernity, genetics and risk

The central message of this chapter has so far been that the experience of ill-health, whatever its cause and however it is manifest, involves individuals and groups in negotiating their own social identity and those of others. Being 'sick' defines the sufferer as being 'different', either because the disorder poses some kind of threat to their 'normal' identity, or because it requires them to withdraw to some degree from the range of activities that are socially defined as 'normal'. These negotiations require sufferers and those who they encounter to negotiate different kinds of knowledge, and to work through different kinds of institutional systems. They thus have a 'career', a trajectory which carries them through different kinds of social identity. Some of these identities have a long history, and we can trace their experiences through different historical periods and identify a variety of responses to them: but the enormously rapid expansion of biomedical knowledge also means that new kinds of identities are being constructed for those who suffer novel disease states, as these are encountered and named through biomedical science.

Genetics is currently the major focus of scientific development in medicine. The astonishing rapidity of advances in knowledge in this field have profoundly reshaped the possibilities of diagnosis in recent years. In particular, genetic explanations of health and disease have begun to undermine the explanatory power of other models of disease causation in recent years, because all explanations are – to some extent, at least – dependent on events at molecular level. Thus, genetic models of disease have been accommodated within medical rhetoric in the most thoroughgoing way. One commentator has noted that:

> Though it is only one conceptual model, "genetics" is increasingly identified as *the* way to reveal and explain health and disease, normality and abnormality.
>
> (Lippman 1994, p.144)

The extent to which this process permits the medicalization of a whole range of variations in human behaviour and biophysiology has been well understood for some time (Yoxen 1983). In the popular media, genetic testing is increasingly represented as a powerful means of achieving diagnostic certainty, and of obtaining the most basic explanation of a variety of problems. That this is translated in the popular imagination as part of a process of developing certainty about the first causes of those health problems, and thus of obtaining 'the answer' to those problems, is therefore not surprising. But what is important here is the extent to which such certainty implies powerful means of attributing a psychosocial identity to those who suffer different kinds of health problems with a genetic basis.

As we have already noted, much work has suggested the detrimental effects on the patient of labelling, and the iatrogenic effects of medical knowledge and practice. But this runs counter to the extent to which diagnostic labels are sought and frequently welcomed by lay users of health services. Suzy's experience of back pain, described earlier in this chapter, is an example of this. Similarly, Becker and Nachtigall (1992) have shown how couples experiencing fertility problems actively constituted these as disease states, and sought medical attention for them, assuming a normative status for childbearing. There is thus an inconsistency between anxieties about the intrusion of medical explanatory models into new domains of social life, and concerns over the continuing incapacity of medical practice to deal with unsolved problems around the causes and cures of specific problems. The growth of genetic medicine offers a case in point, but at present we know remarkably little about the impact of ideas about genetics and risk on individuals and groups.

Clinical genetics sits at a point where the diagnostic imperative that underpins the eagerness of individuals to apply a biomedical explanatory model to their health state, and the rapidly expanding universe of medical knowledge and practice meet. The sheer complexity of new knowledge about genetics, however, means that it needs to be communicated to the patient in a slightly different way to medical knowledge derived from older specialisms that are better understood by the lay population. In this context, genetic counselling has emerged as a subspeciality that is organized around a new context for the transmission of new types of information to the patient. The most important aspect of this is that the very identity of the patient has been redefined. Where, throughout the history of medicine the patient has been constituted as the substantive instance of a disease, and diagnosis has been concerned with identifying the course of a disease in an individual person, genetics diagnosis extends beyond the individual. This involves a new kind of work for the doctor – extending and understanding the probable causes and effects of a disease across kin networks. The patient is thus no longer a discrete individual, but is now much more amorphous. Similarly, the doctor is now concerned with attributing a new kind of social identity – a **genetic** identity – which may have ramifications far beyond the bounds of an individual clinical encounter. This brings with it new dilemmas for the doctor: and new kinds of problems for families. The evidence available to us suggests that genetic medicine and genetic knowledge pose a whole range of risks to kin networks. We can see this in the interview extract produced below, which is drawn from a study which explored the ways that lay users of a genetic counselling service interpreted the medical knowledge it imparted to them.

> My dad is from a very old generation, he's the boss. He makes all the decisions, and I think he put a lot of stick on [my mother] saying, "it's all your fault", and that. It could turn out that it's all his fault. But my sisters (. . .) have been upset, and said a few times, "it's all your fault", to my mum. Which has made her upset, (. . .) There have been a few words said, I think. The general tone, the atmosphere, when they are speaking to my mum, as though it's her fault.
>
> (Chapple and May 1996, p.169)

In this case, the cause for concern is the transmission of a simple inherited defect called Fragile X syndrome. Genes, of course, are morally neutral: but what is at issue here is the way in which they are interpreted in lay settings. For the mother, who has three daughters of childbearing age, the possibility of transmitting a genetic defect that will damage their children is a horrifying prospect. But, in fact, subsequent tests revealed that she was not the carrier. Her husband was 'to blame'. The important point, of course, is that no-one is 'to blame' for inherited defects. But in this case, as in other kinds of illness experience, interpretation derives not simply from apparently neutral and asocial scientific knowledge, but from concepts that relate personal misfortune to moral categories. Berry (1994) noted that the categorization of moral responsibility for inherited defects often falls to women; and Finch (1989) observes that:

> Gender also represents a principle through which different treatment is filtered: you treat male and female relatives differently, in many cases (. . .). Important distinctions are made, even within the group of people that you treat differently, about what kind of different treatment is appropriate.
>
> (Finch 1989, p.234)

Underpinning debates about the impact of genetic knowledge on lay experiences are important ideas about risk. The understanding of risks has become one of the major research enterprises in medical sociology in recent years. Parsons and Atkinson (1992), for example, have explored lay constructs of genetic risk in Duchenne muscular dystrophy. Commenting on their study, Gabe (1995) observes that it shows how:

> women live with the risk of Duchenne Muscular Dystrophy and how awareness of being "at risk" is related to critical junctures in the life course, such as the beginning of courtship, or being in a stable relationship and wanting to have children.
>
> (Gabe 1995, p.8)

What is crucial about 'risk' therefore is not its presence as an abstract concept, but rather its relationship with the kinds of extended social contexts that we have alluded to elsewhere in this chapter. Lay constructs of risk are part of everyday life, but they gather importance and concrete meaning when they are placed in the context of key life events. Their lay interpretations, therefore, need to be situated against the availability and accessibility of knowledge that individuals derive from wider sources.

In their everyday worlds, individuals confront such knowledge not simply in isolated interactions with others, but through relationships with social institutions that represent abstract or expert systems of knowledge (Giddens 1991). To turn again to Gabe's essay we find that:

> The depth of ambivalence or alienation which people feel towards experts and risk management institutions in turn relates to a recognition that we now live in a "risk society" (. . .); that is one that is increasingly vulnerable to major sociotechnological dislocation and social interdependency. Social and economic processes have created global nuclear, chemical, genetic and ecological hazards for which there is no satisfactory aftercare. These structural features reinforce the need for trust in expert authority at the very time that increasing reflexivity and a growing recognition [of] the indeterminate status of knowledge about risk work to undermine it.
>
> (Gabe 1995, p.11).

The key point here is that lay definitions of health and illness, and of the health risks that circulate in complex industrial societies are mediated to individuals not simply through their own experiences, but through received ideas about the potential hazards that confront us. So lay experiences of illness need to be understood not simply in the context of individualized accounts of the personal meaning of illness, but also through their relation to ideas that circulate in abstract bodies of knowledge.

Summary

In a sense, at the end of this chapter, we have arrived at the point at which we began in Chapter 7. That is, we are situating our account at the point where everyday ideas about health and illness interact with professional constructs. In each of the case studies that we have discussed here, the engagement of the sufferers with professional definitions of illness, derived from a variety of sources, have been crucial to forming the bedrock of their experience of illness. It makes no sense to isolate the sufferer from the kinds of knowledge that they draw upon to define their state of health: Bob, for instance, found psychological notions about the aetiology of disease to be of real practical utility in defining the origins and manifestation of Peyronnie's disease; while later in the chapter we have shown how ideas about 'blame' were dismantled by a family suffering from a genetic disorder through genetic testing.

What a sociological perspective on experiences of ill-health does bring to the health professional, therefore, is a way of understanding the impact of a disorder **and** its professional definition, on the sufferer. Professional practice, whether by nurses or others, brings the sufferer into contact – and sometimes conflict – with new kinds of self-identity, new notions of who she or he is in relation to others, and new ways of forming those relationships.

References

Becker G. and Nachtigall R. (1992) 'Born to be a mother': the cultural construction of risk in infertility treatment in the US. *Social Science and Medicine* 39, 507–518.

Berry A. (1994) Genetic counselling: a medical perspective, in Clarke A. (ed.) *Genetic Counselling: practice and principles*. London, Routledge.

Bury M. (1982) Chronic illness as biographical disruption. *Sociology of Health and Illness* 5, 168–195.

Chapple A. and May C. (1996) Genetic knowledge and family relation-ships: two case studies. *Health and Social Care in the Community* 4, 166–171.

Chapple A., Ling M. and May C. (1995) Menorrhagia: women's need for equity in NHS treatment. *Reproductive Health Matters* 9, 132–137.

Finch J. (1989) *Family Obligations and Social Change.* Cambridge, Polity Press.

Gabe J. (1995) Health, medicine and risk: the need for a sociological approach, in Gabe J. (ed.) *Medicine, Health and Risk: sociological approaches.* Oxford, Blackwell.

Giddens A. (1991) *Modernity and Self-Identity.* Cambridge, Polity Press.

Goffman E. (1961) *Stigma.* Harmondsworth, Penguin.

Goffman E. (1963) *Stigma: notes on the management of spoiled identity.* Harmondsworth, Middlesex, Penguin.

Good B. (1994) *Medicine Rationality and Experience: an anthropological perspective.* Cambridge, Cambridge University Press.

Hillary R. (1941) *The Last Enemy.* Harmondsworth, Penguin.

Karp D. (1996) *Speaking of Sadness: depression, disconnection and the meanings of illness.* Oxford, Oxford University Press.

Lewis S. (1995) A search for meaning: making sense of depression. *Journal of Mental Health* 4, 369–382.

Lippman A. (1994) Prenatal testing and screening, in Clarke A. (ed.) *Genetic Counselling: practice and principles.* London, Routledge.

Lupton D. (1995) *The Imperative of Health.* London, Sage.

Lupton D. (1994) *Moral Threats and Dangerous Desires: AIDS in the news media.* London, Taylor and Francis.

Mechanic D. (1968) *Medical Sociology.* New York, Free Press.

Parsons E. and Atkinson P. (1992) Lay constructions of genetic risk. *Sociology of Health and Illness* 14, 437–455.

Parsons T. (1951) *The Social System.* Cambridge, Cambridge University Press.

Pinder R. (1993) *The Management of Chronic Illness: patient and doctor perspectives on Parkinson's disease.* Basingstoke, Macmillan.

Scambler G. (1989) *Epilepsy.* London, Routledge.

Shilts R. (1990) *And the Band Played On.* London, Pelican.

Thorogood N. (1993) Caribbean home remedies and their importance for black women's health in Britain, in Beattie A. *et al* (eds) *Health and Wellbeing: a reader.* Buckingham, Open University Press.

Turner B.S. (1995) *Medical Power and Social Knowledge,* 2nd edn. London, Sage.

Williams G. and Popay J. (1994) Lay knowledge and the privilege of experience, in Gabe J. *et al.* (eds) *Challenging Medicine.* London, Routledge.

Yoxen E. (1983) Constructing genetic disease, in Wright P. and Treacher A. (eds) *The Problem of Medical Knowledge.* Edinburgh, Edinburgh University Press.

9

Death

The denial of death

> Death is now perceived as socially unacceptable or forbidden. Death is dirty and
> indecent, an unfair violation of life which should be preventable . . .. Death is to
> be removed or hidden from social view. Dying is displaced from the home to
> institutions . . .. Mourning is restrained and often almost perfunctory.
>
> (Corr, 1993)

> The announcements that death is taboo and that our society denies death
> continue, yet death is more and more talked of.
>
> (Walter, 1994)

According to Simpson (1987), death is a 'badly kept secret'. Such an
unmentionable topic that there are now thousands of books in print
announcing that we are ignoring the subject of death. How then do
we make sense of the persistence of the view that our society is 'death
denying' (Becker 1973), and what evidence is there to support such
an assertion?

In 1955, Gorer wrote a short article entitled the 'the pornography of
death', in it he argued that death could no longer be discussed openly,
it had become clandestine, as secret as sex was to the Victorians.
Death as a natural process had become unmentionable and yet
violent death played an increasing part in the fantasies offered to
mass audiences. This 'pornography of death' was the price that our
culture paid for distancing itself from natural death.

Gorer's article was followed by many similar arguments, most
notably in the work of Aries (1981) who used selective historical
documents and artefacts to argue that death had become hidden in
contemporary society. According to Aries, the nineteenth century was
the 'beginning of the lie'. Prior to this period, everyone died in public.

The death of a man still solemnly altered the space and time of a social group that could be extended to include the whole community.

Aries noted with approval the elaborate mourning rituals that accompanied 'traditional' death and in particular, that :

Women in mourning were invisible under their crepe and voluminous black veils.

In contrast according to Aries, society now ignores death and:

everything in town goes on as if nobody had died any more.

Aries has been criticized for his sweeping generalizations about whole epochs of European history and also for the fact that he writes exclusively about the 'dying man' and the wealthy dying man at that. Traditional society paid scant attention to the death of the poor who are probably treated with more dignity and respect today. Furthermore, traditional mourning practices say as much about the subordination of women as about contemporary attitudes to death. Recent mass movements such as those following the Dunblane massacre and the death of Diana, Princess of Wales, suggests that new mourning rituals have arisen to replace the more formal rituals of the past.

Writers such as Aries romanticized pre-modern death, seeing it as characterized by an openness and emotional accompaniment which has been contrasted with the bleakness and isolation of modern death. These ideas about the 'denial of death' provided a rallying cry for movements such as the hospice movement, which sought to reform the care of the dying and bereaved. In the nineteenth century nurse reformers presented the image of Sarah Gamp as a lower-class drunkard, incompetent and dangerous. They sought to replace her with a sanitized, Christianized and disciplined workforce. They harked back to a mediaeval past in which nursing was a sacred duty, in order to justify their reforms. Similarly, the movement to humanize death which Lofland (1978) has dubbed the 'happy death' movement hark back to an idealized past and contrast it with the horrors of modern death. The image of the hospital death, alone, afraid, in pain and surrounded by machinery is contrasted with traditional death within the bosom of the family.

Contemporary historians have reassessed the myth of Sarah Gamp, arguing that it was a stereotype convenient to the reformers of the time, but not strictly accurate (Dingwall, Rafferty and Webster 1988). Perhaps the 'denial of death' will be similarly recognized as a myth in years to come.

Certainly, for a 'taboo' subject, death is overwhelmingly present (Walter 1991). Gorer argued that the ever-growing fantasies of death portrayed in the media were pornographic because they were devoid of humanity and emotion. Yet much media coverage of death deals precisely with these emotional issues offering a commentary on the grief of the dying and bereaved (Walter, Littlewood and Pickering 1995). The death of Diana, Princess of Wales provoked an outpouring of discussions about such feelings within the media. Walter *et al.* described this media coverage as 'emotional invigilation'. When dealing with death, popular culture is preoccupied with acceptable and unacceptable expressions of suffering and grief. Emotional expression is approved, but not too much, and we must show we care but we must also be brave. The death of Princess Diana offered enormous scope to the media in their discussions of the proper reactions of the Royal family, politicians, the public and even of their own feelings.

So brave, grief stricken William and Harry hold back the tears

The Duchess has lost someone she has always considered a sister. There are no words to describe the pain in her heart

We are a nation today in a state of shock, in mourning, in grief that is so deeply painful for us

I am crying as I write this . . . I cannot believe Diana is dead

(*Daily Mirror*, 1997)

According to Walter *et al.* such preoccupation's reflect a new uncertainty about how to act and feel in the face of suffering and death in that prescribed mourning rituals have disappeared. Hardly, though a 'pornography of death'.

Others have argued that death is both present and absent in modern society. Blauner (1966) suggested that better life expectancy meant that death in the prime of life is now the exception rather than the rule. When deaths from infectious diseases were prevalent, death touched the lives of everyone. Social life was threatened by the deaths of younger people who still had important social roles. Mourning rituals were necessary to restore social equilibrium because death often disrupted the social order. Now that most people are old when they die, their death affects few people as they have already relinquished their social roles. Furthermore, with rapid social change, the skills and knowledge of the old are no longer seen as a valuable resource to be handed on to a younger generation. Instead, the old are seen as obsolete, 'past their sell by date'. The old, it is argued, are socially dead before they are biologically dead (Sudnow, 1967). Social death occurs when an individual is no longer an 'active agent in the social world' (Mulkay 1993) and comes to be treated as a non-person.

These ideas suggest that death is no longer a problem for society, merely a problem for the individual who is dying or bereaved. Social rituals and support have broken down and individuals are isolated, left to make their own way through this personal crisis.

The sequestration of death

We have seen that it is argued that death is both 'present' and 'absent' in contemporary culture (Mellor 1993). It is necessary for individuals to some extent to ignore death in order to commit themselves to everyday life. Death can call into question the world-building activities of individuals and a failure to deal with death adequately can threaten our individual and collective sense of meaning.

> Individuals have to face extreme terrors of personal meaningless – but the social order as a whole becomes vulnerable to a collapse into chaos with a more widespread attendant, loss of meaning and order.
>
> (Mellor 1993)

This concurs with Berger's (1967) view that:

> Every human society is in the last resort men (and women) banded together in the face of death.

A major concern for some authors is the decline in religious values which offered a communal response to death. Secularization is assumed to be an accomplished fact and the absence of religious explanations and rituals is seen to lead to private anxiety and anomie. According to Turner (1991):

> We are exposed to the material world of commodities objects and bodies without the intervening shield of religious meanings. The death of God has left us literally and culturally naked.

Giddens (1991), has noted that a particular feature of contemporary society (an era he describes as 'high modernity'), is a concern with issues of self-identity. A variety of therapies and self-help guides help us to create a positive self-image and sense of self. An important part of the cultivation of self-identity is the cultivation of the body. Consumer culture places enormous emphasis on products to enhance the appearance and well-being of the body and increasing importance is placed on the body as constitutive of the self (Mellor 1993). Sinhalese society individuals of the Buddhist faith meditate on the putrefaction of the body as a religious duty to remind them of the transience of their earthly existence (Obeyesekere 1989). In high modernity, bodily fitness is cultivated to ward off thoughts of death and decay, lest such thoughts bring with them the onslaught of the nightmare (Berger and Luckman 1967).

Thus, many contemporary sociologists see us building a world of meanings in which death is distant or absent, something that happens only to other people. In such a world, the dying and bereaved are isolated. Elias (1985) argues that 'civilizing processes' that have shaped our society place a high value on privacy and emotional reserve. Thus, it is no longer possible to speak to the dying and bereaved and they are condemned to unalterable loneliness.

For Mellor (1993), it is this 'privatization of meaning' which has led to the 'sequestration' of death. The dying are hidden away in institutions and isolated from human contact. Even hospices are seen as contributing to this process by Mellor, despite the high value placed on home care by the hospice movement and the fact that 50% of their patients are discharged home to die. In contrast to this view, Seale (1995a) argues that our society places a high value on emotional accompaniment at the time of death. His study of those who had died alone showed that for survivors, dying alone was seen as a threatening and untoward event for which they had to account and atone.

The rationalization of death

We have seen therefore, that there is an influential discourse that argues that death has become hidden, that we have become a death-denying society and that this discourse remains influential despite much evidence to contradict it.

For other commentators, contemporary public discourses about death have not ceased but changed. We have moved from a religious to a scientific and bureaucratic treatment of death. At the same time as a decline in mourning rituals occurred, the surveillance of death by the state became increasingly important. A massive new discourse arose centred around the certification of death, the post-mortem and the coroners' court (Armstrong 1987).

Throughout the nineteenth century, there was a vocal debate on the disposal of the dead and accounting for death became vital to the government of populations. Modern social institutions are predicated on actuarial calculations of the risk of mortality. Where would epidemiology, public health or indeed the insurance industry be without mortality statistics? Accounting for death became a medicolegal discourse which located death and disease within the human body. The discipline of pathology looked for explanations of death within the corpse and the social organization of death came to be framed around this physicalist and individualist explanation of death (Prior 1989).

Modern techniques of surveillance of the corpse were not achieved without resistance. A belief in the resurrection of the dead led many to oppose the dissection of corpses. Before the 1832 Anatomy Act, dissection was part of the punishment reserved for convicted felons and there was great public concern about the growth of grave robbery to supply the expanding medical schools with corpses. The 1832 Anatomy Act permitted the bodies of paupers to be used for dissection. Thus, poverty rather than crime was hereafter punished by dismemberment (Richardson 1989). It is important not to sentimentalize the past. Writers like Gorer and Aries have noted with approval that in Victorian times the corpse remained at home in the front parlour until the funeral. Richardson notes that the poor often kept the corpse at home until it began to rot in order to ensure that their loved one was in an unfit state for the pathologist's scalpel.

Prior's study of the certification of death shows how the medicolegal management of death came to individualize explanations of the cause of death. Until the end of the nineteenth century, the vocabulary of causation linked the physical body to the social body. Early reports of coroners and the Registrar General included reference to the price of food and fuel, levels of pauperism and the climate. In the nineteenth century you could still officially die of poverty, neglect or 'unskilful medical treatment'. Gradually social factors and human agency were erased from accounts of death, so that by the late twentieth century, a victim of violence in Belfast is recorded as having died from 'bruising and oedema of the brain associated with fractures of the skull' .

Adams (1993) argues that this rationalist discourse about death is also a masculinist discourse. The social management of death has been transferred from the home and the community to the hospital, coroner and funeral director. At the same time care of the corpse has transferred from women to men. Adams charts the decline of the female neighbourhood 'layer out', whose activities were part of a network of mutual support. Laying out was part of a 'rationality of care' within the domestic setting. These women have been replaced by the male mortician and funeral director who view the corpse as an impersonal work object. Smith (1992) notes that performing last offices is often used by nurses as a point of closure in a caring relationship and Kiger (1994) similarly found that nurses accorded significance to last offices as the 'last thing' they could do for their patient. As a largely female profession, nurses are attempting to deliver a caring service within an institution which is founded on a masculinist discourse of scientific rationality.

Hafferty (1988) sees the treatment of the corpse as an object, as an important part of the emotional socialization of medical students. Learning to respond to the dissection of a human corpse with detachment is also learning the 'feeling rules' (Hochschild 1983) of medicine. The corpse must be viewed as a learning tool and object of manipulation rather than as a formerly living human being. The informal culture of medical students abounds with tales in which medical students dismember human corpses in order to shock an outsider. This oral culture reinforces medicines 'feeling rules' and draws a sharp boundary between medical and lay culture. Hafferty suggests that there is a danger that feeling rules that operate to distance medical students from the emotional consequence of dissecting patients will 'bleed' into other areas, encouraging emotional detachment from living patients.

Baumann (1987) and Ritzer (1996) have argued that the scientific rationalist discourse about death found its most complete expression in the Nazi Holocaust. Death and killing were bureaucratized and medicalized. Doctors and nurses attended the railway sidings at Auschwitz to sort the inmates of incoming trains into those fit to survive and those for disposal in the gas chambers. For them the Jews had already attained 'thing-like' status, they were socially dead.

According to Baumann:

> the technical-administrative success of the Holocaust was due in part to the skilful utilization of "moral sleeping pills" made available by modern bureaucracy and modern technology.

Seidelman (1991) suggests that medicine is still founded on a rationalist discourse which seeks to divide those who are fit to live from those who are not. The discourse of rationing, cost-effectiveness, 'health gains' and quality adjusted life-years (QALYS) is built on the railway sidings of Auschwitz. A recent expression of this discourse is the debate over the 'high cost of dying' (Scitovsky 1994). US statistics showing high medical expenditure in the last months of life have led to calls to curtail treatment to reduce cost. The concept of 'medical futility' is employed to back calls for cost containment in the care of the dying. Calls to curtail treatment of the dying treat the dying as already socially dead. Similarly, the rationalist discourse about euthanasia seeks to hasten biological death so that it is coterminous with social death. As the medical profession and the courts increasingly debate whether individual lives are worth living, some sociologists wish us to remember the historical antecedents of such discourse.

Revisiting the 'denial of death'

One answer to the question 'Are we a death denying society?' has been that death has been subject to unprecedented scrutiny, but that a scientific, rationalist discourse has replaced a religious and personal one. Thus, according to Armstrong (1987), the truth about death has been sought by interrogation of the physical body rather than in the words of the dying man.

A more recent view is that death has been rediscovered largely through what Lofland has described as the 'happy death' movement. As Aries (1981) has noted:

> Shown the door by society, death is coming back in by the window.

Walter (1994) suggests that the 'revival of death' reflects wider cultural changes, in particular the 'expressive revolution' of the 1960s. The expressivist model considers that if emotions are not displayed, a whole range of pathologies will follow. Thus, it follows that people **ought** to express emotions particularly negative ones. Walter links the 'expressive' revolution to moves to 'subjectify' the patient. Expressivism implies an extension of the professional gaze:

> If medicine in the Age of Reason gazed upon the body and upon the corpse, whole person medicine today gazes upon the psyche.
>
> (Walter 1994)

Linked to the culture of expressivism has been a renewed interest in religion. As we noted in the discussion on secularization in an earlier chapter, the assumption that religious belief has declined is perhaps overstated and the revival of religious beliefs in a number of segments of society is well documented.

The 'happy death' movement has sought to invest death with new meaning and these values find their expression in the concept of the 'good death'. The good death is one where there is awareness, acceptance and discussion of death. Sociologists have played an important part in constructing the concept of the 'Good Death' and we will now turn our attention to the way in which sociologists have influenced and informed contemporary developments in caring for the dying.

Communication and awareness of dying

An important goal of the hospice movement has been to improve communication with the dying. Studies in this field have criticized communication with dying patients and accused health professionals of a lack of commitment and skill (Ford, Fallowfield and Lewis 1996).

Much of our understanding of communication with the dying has derived from the work of Glaser and Strauss in 1965. In their work with the dying in San Francisco hospitals they found a number of 'awareness contexts'. In 'closed awareness' the truth was kept from the patient. 'Suspicion' awareness exists when the patient tried unsuccessfully to extract the truth from family and carers. 'Mutual pretence' existed when both sides pretended to be unaware of the truth. In 'open awareness' the truth was shared between patient, family and staff.

Glaser and Strauss criticized the high levels of closed awareness in their study associating it with unhappiness and isolation. Their work has been used widely to argue for more honesty with dying patients and to promote the emotional accompaniment of patients in their journey towards death.

Recent surveys suggest that there is now much more openness on the part of health professionals dealing with the dying. Williams (1989) suggests that in the USA it is now the rule to tell patients of their diagnosis rather than the exception. In the UK, the approach has been rather more cautious with doctors emphasizing the patient's wish to know as a deciding factor. Seale (1991) found that the increased openness with patients was largely found in the treatment of cancer patients. Cancer patients are much more likely to be told the truth than patients dying of other conditions. This does not necessarily reflect the certainty of their prognosis because patients dying of other conditions were often not told, even when death was expected.

There have been a number of criticisms of the concept of 'awareness contexts', perhaps most importantly they imply that doctors have certain knowledge that they can choose to impart to the patient or not. This underestimates the uncertainty of diagnosis and prognosis in many conditions. Schou (1993) suggests that dying is an ambiguous concept and that 'there is no facile boundary between the end of mainstream treatment and the beginning of dying'. In her study of oncology units, there was a general preference for openness with patients, yet this sat uncomfortably with the orientation of these units towards curative treatment. Oncology units tried to promote an upbeat image in which the battle against cancer was one that they could be seen to be winning and yet in reality most patients receiving active treatment had scant chance of a cure. Timmermans (1994) suggests that uncertainty may be a strategy used by patients and staff alike to maintain hope. By contrast, in critical care, Harvey (1996) found that staff constantly struggled to achieve certainty and control in what were often highly unpredictable situations. Thus, the concept of open awareness remains problematical despite its wide acceptance.

Nursing the dying

As we have noted in previous chapters, nurses have come to view the nurse–patient relationship as central to their endeavours. Nurses caring for the dying talk at length of the importance of their role in communicating with the dying. Ironically, this view is not always shared by patients. Seale (1991) found that patients saw doctors as the most important source of information and family and friends as the most important source of emotional support. Mayer (1987) reported that cancer patients rated technical competence as the most important component of nursing, whereas nurses rated expressive activities such as listening to the patient most highly. James (1992) in her study of hospice nursing suggested that caring was composed of physical labour, emotional labour and organization. It may be that patients are telling us that physical and emotional labour are inseparable and that we cannot privilege one above another. The procedure of last offices is a good example of the interdependence of physical and emotional labour and the abandonment of this task by nurses in many hospitals can be seen as symbolic of the 'disembodiment' of the patient by the nurse.

Humanizing death

We have seen that the hospice movement has changed attitudes to the dying in recent times, particularly in relation to the care of cancer patients. The rationalization of death tended to remove death from the care and control of the family and community to bureaucratic institutions and according to Adams (1993) represented a 'defeminization' of death. Seale (1995b) suggests that the new discourses about death promoted by the hospice movement present death as an emotional and spiritual journey and offer a new form of 'heroic death' in which the individual can demonstrate courage and a 'beatific state' in the face of death. This, says Seale, represents particularly feminine heroics with its emphasis on emotional expression and self sacrifice. We can thus talk of a 'refeminization' of death.

Positive though this humanization of death may be, we must note its limitations. The 'heroic script' is most available to younger patients dying from cancer and AIDS. The hospice movement has had little impact on those dying from other conditions. A particular change noted in Seale's study has been the increasing numbers of elderly people dying in private residential homes and palliative care and emotional accompaniment in their journey towards death are remote. For these people, death has not been humanized. These are the 'disadvantaged dying'.

According to Seale (1995b):

> Those who are in extreme old age . . . the demented and the institutionalized, have much less opportunity to strike an heroic pose, but are more frequently portrayed as dribbling, undignified figures, waiting for death as a release from life. The lives and deaths of these individuals have become the horror stories of our time.

Until we recognize our responsibility to all who are dying, the 'happy death' movement will be unable to claim that it has truly humanized death.

References

Adams S. (1993) A gendered history of the social management of death in Foleshill, Coventry, during the interwar years, in Clark D. (ed) *The Sociology of Death: theory, culture, practice*. Cambridge, Blackwell.

Aries P. (1981) *The Hour of our Death*. London, Allen Lane.

Armstrong D. (1987) Silence and truth in death and dying. *Social Science and Medicine*. 8, 651–657.

Baumann Z. (1987) *Modernity and the Holocaust*. Oxford, Polity.

Becker E. (1973) *The Denial of Death*. New York, Free Press.

Berger P. (1967) *The Sacred Canopy: elements of a sociological theory of religion*. New York, Doubleday.

Berge, P. and Luckman T. (1967) *The Social Construction of Reality; a treatise in the sociology of knowledge*. London, Penguin.

Blauner R. (1966) Death and social structure. *Psychiatry* 29, 378–394.

Corr C. (1993) Death in modern society, in Doyle D. (ed) *Oxford Textbook of Palliative Medicine*. Oxford, Oxford University Press.

Dingwall R., Rafferty A. and Webster C. (1988) *An Introduction of the Social History of Nursing*. London, Routledge.

Elias N. (1985) *The Loneliness of the Dying*. London, Routledge.

Ford S., Fallowfield L. and Lewis S. (1996) Doctor patient interactions in oncology. *Social Science and Medicine*. 42(11), 1511–1519.

Giddens A. (1991) *Modernity and Self Identity*. Oxford, Polity.

Glaser B. and Strauss A. (1965) *Awareness of Dying*. Chicago, Aldine.

Gorer G. (1955) The Pornography of Death. *Encounter* October.

Hafferty F. (1988) Cadaver stories and the emotional socialisation of medical students. *Journal of Health and Social Behaviour* 29, 344–356.

Harvey J. (1996) Achieving the indeterminate: accomplishing degrees of certainty in life and death situations. *Sociological Review* 44, 78–98.

Hochschild A. (1983) *The Managed Heart: commercialisation of human feeling*. Berkeley, University of California Press.

James N. (1992) Care = organisation + physical labour + emotional labour. *Sociology of Health and Illness* 14(4), 488–509.

Kiger A. (1994) Student nurses' involvement with death: the image and the experience. *Journal of Advanced Nursing* 20, 679–686.

Lofland L. (1978) *The Craft of Dying: the modern face of death.* Beverley Hills, Sage.

Mayer D. (1987) Oncology nurses' versus cancer patients' perceptions of nurse caring behaviours: a replication. *Oncology Nurses Forum.* 14(3), 48–52.

Mellor P. (1993) Death in high modernity: the contemporary presence and absence of death, In Clark, D. (ed.) *The Sociology of Death: theory, culture, practice.* Cambridge, Blackwell.

Mulkay M. (1993) 'Social Death in Britain', in Clark D. (ed). *The Sociology of Death: theory, culture, practice.* Cambridge, Blackwell.

Obeyesekere G. (1989) Despair and Recovery, in Sinhala medicine and religion: an anthropologists meditations, in Sullivan L.E. (ed.) *Healing and Restoring Health and Medicine in the World's Religious Traditions.* Macmillan, New York and London.

Prior L. (1989) *The Social Organisation of Death: medical discourse and social practices in Belfast.* London, Macmillan.

Richardson R. (1989) *Death, Dissection and the Destitute.* London, Penguin.

Ritzer G. (1996) *The McDonaldisation of Society.* California, Pine Forge Press.

Schou K. (1993) Awareness contexts and the construction of dying in the cancer treatment setting: 'micro' and 'macro' levels in narrative analysis', in Clark D. (ed.) *The Sociology of Death: theory, culture, practice.* Cambridge, Blackwell.

Scitovsky A. (1994). The 'high cost of dying' revisited. *Millbank Memorial Fund Quarterly* 72(4), 561–591.

Seale C. (1991). Communication and awareness about death: a study of a random sample of dying people. *Social Science and Medicine* 32(8), 943–952.

Seale C. (1995a) Dying alone. *Sociology of Health and Illness* 17(3), 376–392.

Seale C. (1995b) Heroic death. *Sociology* 29(4), 597–613.

Seidelman W. (1991) Medical selection: Auschwitz antecedents and effluent. *International Journal of Health Services* 21(3), 401–415.

Simpson M. (1987) *Dying, death and grief: a critical bibliography.* University of Philadelphia Press.

Smith P. (1992). *The Emotional Labour of Nursing.* London, Macmillan.

Sudnow D. (1967). *Passing On: the social organisation of dying.* Englewood Cliffs, Prentice Hall.

Timmermans S. (1994). Dying of awareness: the theory of awareness contexts revisited. *Sociology of Health and Illness* 16(3), 322–339.

Turner B. (1991) *Religion and Social Theory.* London, Sage.

Walter T. (1991) Modern death – taboo or not taboo. *Sociology* 22(2), 293–310.

Walter T. (1994) *The Revival of Death.* London, Routledge.

Walter T., Littlewood J. and Pickering M. (1995) Death in the News: the public invigilation of private emotion. *Sociology* 29(4), 579–596

Williams R. (1989) Awareness and control of dying: some paradoxical trends in public opinion. *Sociology of Health and Illness* 11(3), 201–212.

Afterword

We hope that in this book we have given you, the reader, more than a useful textbook that fits the demands of the course that you are doing, and perhaps the essay or dissertation that you are writing. We hope that we have also introduced you to a discipline that is intrinsically interesting: fundamentally, sociology is about the circumstances that people find themselves in, about why they speak and act in the ways that they do, and about the ways in which their lives are shaped and organized by powerful social forces and institutions. As a discipline, it seeks to comprehend our common experience of living in 'society' as well as the differences between us. Sociology thus brings explanatory models (theories) of social behaviour, and techniques through which those models can be developed and tested (research methods), to bear on those social forces and institutions in a way that helps us to understand how our live are shaped and organized. If we can understand those things clearly, then perhaps we can change them for the better.

Just as nursing increasingly seeks to understand the patient holistically, so sociology is focused on more than the individual instance of a particular event or illness. As sociologists, we want to understand how and why nursing has taken the path that it has, and how that path might in turn affect the future of the profession. Equally, we want to know how ordinary people and their families manage the experience of ill-health, and how they construct these experiences. This is not just knowledge for the sake of knowing, however. Sociological research has been at the forefront of changing our ideas about how health care might be organized in ways that people find more helpful. Earlier in this book, for example, we observed the impact that sociological research and writing has had on changing attitudes and services around antenatal care and childbirth. Sociological research on the occupational socialization of student nurses played an important part in rethinking nurse training too.

In reviewing the contents of this book we are struck by the breadth as well as the depth of the discipline of sociology, and by the variety of philosophical positions that may be found within it. Sociology extends from very grand macro-level questions about the nature of society; to much more sharply focused questions about the form that interactions between nurses and their patients take. But it also asks serious questions about what health and disease are, and what nursing is (and might be). As a discipline, it goes beyond individual differences and qualities, or the costs and benefits of particular kinds of services, and tries to locate health and the health professions in their wider context.

Because of this, sociology offers opportunities to develop new and interesting ways of framing nursing knowledge and practice. Perhaps the most obvious example here is the emphasis on qualitative methods that characterize nursing research in the UK. Much of this derives directly from sociological theory and method, and in particular from symbolic interactionism. An important feature of this approach is the degree to which it allows the subjects of nursing research to speak 'directly' as it were to the reader of articles and dissertations. It offers the subject an opportunity to 'tell it like it is' (Melia 1987). Our final point is in relation to this: historically, much sociological research has been about giving voice to the experience of those who are not powerful, or those who are unheard for some other reason. Sociology is thus an **ethical** discipline that contributes to advocacy, as well as understanding. It may not be enough simply to understand why, for example, people with mental health problems or some other illness are stigmatized by the form that their care takes. We might want to do something about it.

Hannah Cooke, Anne Williams and Carl May

Reference

Melia K. (1987) *Learning and Working: the occupational socialisation of student nurses*. London, Tavistock.

Index